AF616284

The Global Eradication of Smallpox

New Perspectives in South Asian History 32

The **New Perspectives in South Asian History** series publishes monographs and other writings on early modern, modern and contemporary history. The volumes in the series cover new ground across a broad spectrum of subjects such as cultural, environmental, medical, military and political history, and the histories of 'marginalised' groups. It includes fresh perspectives on more familiar fields as well as interdisciplinary and original work from all parts of South Asia. It welcomes historical contributions from sociology, anthropology and cultural studies.

The Global Eradication of Smallpox

Edited by

Sanjoy Bhattacharya
Sharon Messenger
The Wellcome Trust Centre
for the History of Medicine
University College London

Orient BlackSwan

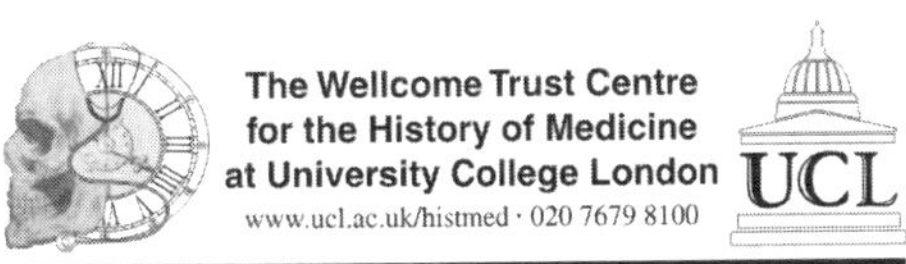

ORIENT BLACKSWAN PRIVATE LIMITED

Registered Office
3-6-752 Himayatnagar, Hyderabad 500 029 (A.P.), India
E-mail: centraloffice@orientblackswan.com

Other Offices
Bangalore, Bhopal, Bhubaneshwar, Chandigarh, Chennai, Ernakulam, Guwahati, Hyderabad, Jaipur, Kolkata, Lucknow, Mumbai, New Delhi, Noida, Patna

First Published 2010

ISBN 978 81 250 3981 5

Typeset by
OSDATA, Hyderabad 500 029
in Bembo (Aldine) 10.5/12.5

Maps cartographed by
Sangam Books (India) Private Limited, Hyderabad

Printed at
Aegean Offset, Greater Noida

Published by
Orient Blackswan Private Limited
1/24 Asaf Ali Road, New Delhi 110 002
E-mail: delhi@orientblackswan.com

The publishers gratefully acknowledge the financial support received for this volume from the Wellcome Trust Centre for the History of Medicine at University College London

Contents

The book is accompanied by a CD containing lectures by

1. Joel G. Breman
2. Larry Brilliant
3. D. A. Henderson
4. Ciro de Quadros
5. Alan Schnur

Figures, Tables and Maps

Introduction

Sanjoy Bhattacharya

The year 1980 witnessed the fulfilment of a goal that many had considered impossible. At the recommendation of an independent commission of experts, the World Health Organization's (WHO) Health Assembly announced the global eradication of smallpox. It was a momentous occasion; in the view of many, with good reason, this was the greatest achievement of global public health in the twentieth century. However, time has taken some shine off the accomplishment. I have encountered, all too often, in idle conversations and more formal presentations of ideas in the form of speeches and writings, the argument that smallpox eradication was easily achieved. According to this interpretation of events, the problems faced by the 'smallpox warriors' were relatively straightforward as the disease did not have animal hosts. Some commentators also argue, quite simplistically, that the work was centred around a strategy of searching for cases, containing infective individuals and vaccinating their immediate contacts with efficacious vaccines.

The situation was always more complicated throughout the course of a long-drawn out global programme. Although it was announced in the late 1950s, the programme really only took off a decade later (after the completion of a series of successful campaigns across West Africa). Notably, its constituent activities took a further ten years to complete in a situation where the South Asian subcontinent and the Horn of Africa threw up a series of unexpected challenges. The mere presence of technological developments—such as the introduction of heat stable freeze dried vaccines, and the so-called bifurcated needle that contributed to vaccinal economy and safety—did not guarantee smallpox eradication. Human agency was an important determinant, since significant efforts had to be made by programme managers within the WHO and national governments to convince field officials to embrace new ideas and technologies. Notably, despite these efforts at persuasion, some people remained indifferent to the calls for the introductions of new operational methods and vaccinal products, choosing to stick to older procedures that they were more comfortable with and often regarded as being more reliable. Other challenges afflicted the campaign as well. Some sections of the target population opposed vaccination, which led to delayed completion of work in some areas and introduced time-consuming negotiations in others. There were, after all, limits to how much pressure the 'smallpox warriors' could impose on local politicians, junior governmental officials and civilians; diplomatic niceties could not be dispensed with altogether and international workers remained wary about stoking violent civilian resistance (force, when it was used, could create lasting resentment, which was recognised as being strategically unhelpful).

Other factors also created difficulties for the global effort at smallpox eradication. Support from within the WHO frameworks in Geneva and the regional offices remained inconstant, and often caused serious financial difficulties for fieldwork; these challenges were only overcome in the 1970s with the assistance provided by a range of donors, like the Swedish and Danish International Development Agencies, the Indian and Bangladeshi governments, and, not least, the Tata industrial consortium in India. To make matters worse—and these trends remained visible right till the end of the campaign—some officials associated to national and local governments continued to oppose the eradication goal, often simply because they considered it misguided. In addition, competing health and financial priorities, alternative epidemiological understandings of smallpox causation and control, and a variety of professional and personal jealousies proved damaging; all these trends stoked doubts amongst bureaucratic and civilian constituencies, which translated into episodes where assistance was refused to teams of 'smallpox warriors'.

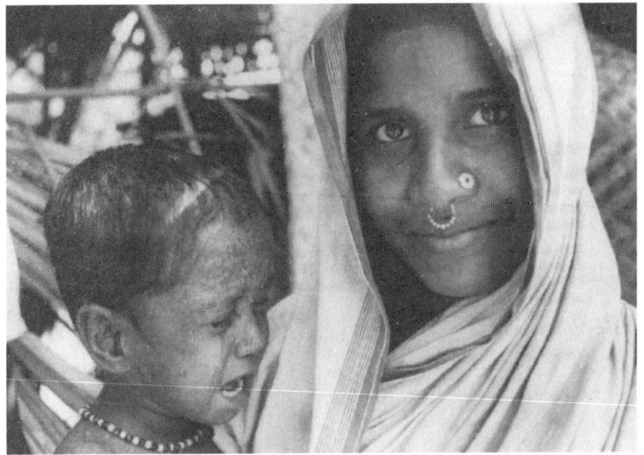

FIGURE I.1: Rahima Banu Begam (born 1973) was the last known person to be infected with naturally occuring *Variola major* smallpox. The case occured on 16 October 1975, when the two-year-old Banu was living in the village of Kuralia on Bhola Island in the district of Barisal, Bangladesh.

Source: © World Health Organization.

There were many positive aspects to the global smallpox eradication programme as well. A large number of participants remember—and cherish—the internationalism that characterised it. For many, including people who have contributed articles to this volume, the campaign allowed a context in which cold war rivalries gradually dissipated, as several officials from the United States (US), erstwhile USSR and countries allied to each learnt to collaborate with and trust each other. It is also worth remembering that many national workers regarded their participation in the project as a career highlight, allowing an intense and productive association with the WHO frameworks; this attitude is well represented by the care and pride with which officials have preserved certificates thanking them for their involvement. There can be little doubt that there was goodwill amongst many 'smallpox warriors', despite differences in nationality, education, race, gender and age. For many young officials, participation in such a global programme led to new career paths, with international and government agencies, non-government organisations (NGOs), universities and charities. A shared goal of saving lives drew many people together in the 1970s and ultimately gave rise to meaningful projects like the Expanded Programme on Immunisation, whose components are widely credited for reducing levels of infantile mortality around the world.

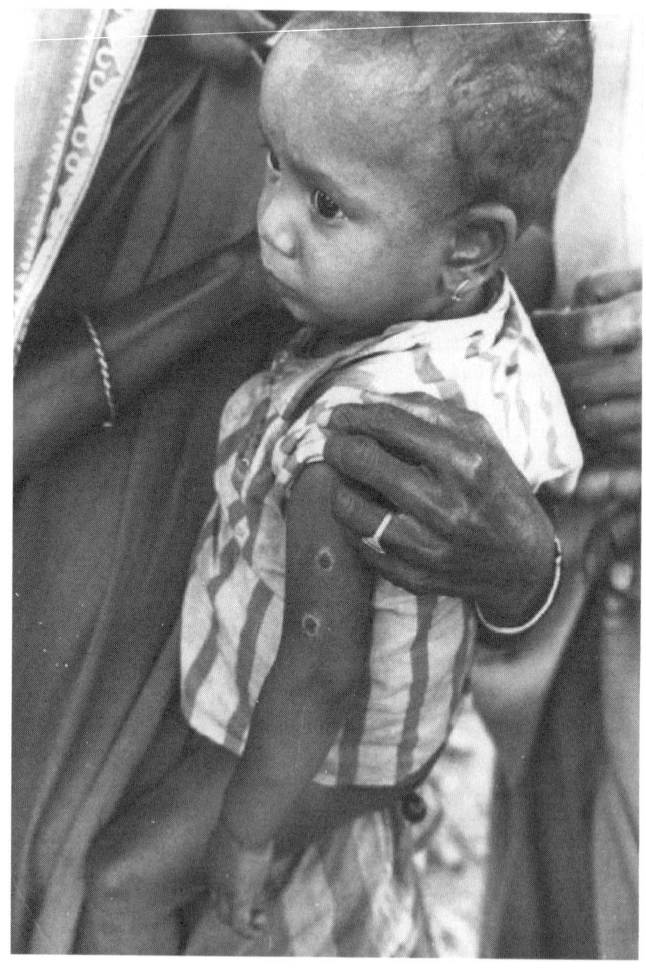

FIGURE I.2: Vaccinated child.

Source: © World Health Organization.

However, all these positives should not be allowed to cloak important intricacies in operational strategy, especially as these are sometimes downplayed or ignored in celebratory treatises. The global smallpox eradication programme, which was composed of several national chapters linked by a series of international accords, was always marked by variations in official and civilian attitudes. Participants had differing visions about the efficacy of plans, and teams were composed of workers with dissimilar levels of ability and commitment. The contours of these attitudinal variations changed over time and place, as there were shifts in the composition of teams and their interactions with various constituencies in national territories and their locales. Also, as several of the articles in this volume remind us, the transfer of ideas about the best means of eradicating smallpox did not flow in one direction. Indeed, the most effective campaigns were generally those that were based on a proactive exchange of ideas between field personnel of different ranks and backgrounds; for this reason, regular meetings between international workers and national counterparts were regarded as being a crucial component of the programme in the 1970s. Many international workers were also able to play another important role—conduits for locally garnered information, which would otherwise have been ignored by those at the apex of national governing structures. Indeed, WHO representatives were often able to put forward ideas presented by junior medical and paramedical staff who were in touch with the social, political and economic realities of specific regions; this frequently ensured that this input was not summarily rejected. The multi-directional flow of ideas—and the resulting impact on field policies—is not always recognised or analysed by chroniclers of smallpox eradication. Yet, these trends need to be studied sensitively and in great depth, so that we are better able to present the many complexities characterising national and local vaccination campaigns.

A spirit of collaboration, in the widest sense, allowed the achievement of the impossible. So, as we celebrate a magnificent achievement in public health cooperation, we should consciously seek to refrain from reducing success to the contributions made by a few individuals associated to specific institutions. These people and organisations could not, on their own, have stamped out the disease; different health agencies worked with each other, with one stepping up to fill the breach whenever another's strength was denuded by constant toil and required time to recover its vitality. Seen from this perspective, a complex association of institutions and people led to the stamping out of variola in its natural form; it is of paramount importance that we do not forget the contributions of the many people who contributed to the triumph. As D. A. Henderson and others deeply involved in running this most remarkable and complicated public health programme remind us, smallpox eradication would have been impossible without the dedication of—and sacrifices made by—a huge number of individuals. It is imperative that we do not forget that a vast majority of these people were drawn from the countries where the final battles against the variola virus were concluded. Many voices need to be remembered and recorded, before they are lost to posterity. But, that is a job for future historians, for whom there remains a lot to study and better understand, not least as efforts continue to be made to learn from past experiences.

This edited volume is a product of two series of public lectures organised by the Wellcome Trust Centre for the History of Medicine at UCL, at 183 Euston Road, London, United Kingdom (UK). Additional support from a Wellcome Trust-funded project grant allowed us to record the lectures and make these the basis of the podcasts that are presented in the attached CD. The editors would like to thank Alan Yabsley and Carole Reeves for all their hard work in producing the CD which accompanies the book. The editors of the book and the CD are deeply grateful to the Wellcome Trust Centre/UCL and the Wellcome Trust for their support. Special thanks should also be made to the staff in the Hyderabad Office of Orient BlackSwan for the production of this volume. In particular the editors would like to thank Osamazaid Rahman for his meticulous copyediting and they would also like to offer generous thanks for the continued hard work and support of Veenu Luthria who has, as always, been a pleasure to work with.

1

The Global Eradication of Smallpox: Historical Perspectives and Future Prospects

D. A. Henderson

Introduction

In 1977, just thirty-three years ago, the last case of smallpox was detected and eradication of the virus was declared. This precipitated increasing interest in undertaking another eradication programme, and a decade later a programme to eradicate poliomyelitis was launched. For more than twenty years now, legions of health workers have struggled towards that goal but, as yet, with no certain end in sight. In frustration as they have failed to deal with this problematic challenge, some have imagined that the smallpox programme was intrinsically straightforward, readily accepted and easily executed. It has been suggested that an acquiescent World Health Assembly unanimously agreed to undertake smallpox eradication; that all countries so feared the disease that all were enthusiastically supportive; that a Geneva-based Central High Command was created to direct field operations; and that armies of vaccinators simply fanned out, and smallpox vanished. The facts could not be more different.

As summarised in this chapter, a programme of smallpox eradication was accepted in the World Health Assembly by the narrowest of margins and only after extended debate; many health

Based on a presentation on 30 May 2007 at the Wellcome Trust Centre for the History of Medicine at UCL.

professionals, including the WHO Director-General, believed the goal to be unattainable; and twice, within the last two years of the programme, it teetered on the verge of catastrophe and possible failure.[1]

The saga of smallpox eradication comprises an extraordinarily diverse array of challenges and successes punctuated by all but insurmountable setbacks, civil wars, floods, famines and refugees. Throughout most of its course, the programme received only tepid support by many key international and national leaders, continuing scarcities of funds and vaccine, rigid bureaucracies, seriously deficient health infrastructures and problems with both communication and transportation. Ultimately, success was finally realised, abetted by a number of notable and unexpected surprises and breakthroughs. All credit is due to imaginative and creative national and international staffs working long hours under inhospitable circumstances in a programme that was anything but simple or straightforward.

There have been several historical accounts of components of the smallpox eradication programme but few by those who were themselves central participants. Such accounts are needed to bring a sense of the realities of the actual implementation of this far-flung venture that involved as many as 120,000 national workers at certain times of the programme, which functioned in some fifty countries but which never had more than 150 international staff in the field at any given time.

Other chapters in this series highlight events in especially important areas. Brazil was an early success and eradication there, only four years after the programme began, permitted certification that the whole of the Western Hemisphere was smallpox free. It was an important impetus to the global effort. A further affirmation that the programme strategy was effective was the eradication of smallpox from all of Western and Central Africa. This occurred less than five years after that programme had begun and included countries that had been among the world's most highly infected and with the most

[1] Material for this chapter has been drawn from two principal sources: F. Fenner, D. A. Henderson, Isao Arita, Z. Jezek and I. D. Ladnyi, *Smallpox and its Eradication* (Geneva: World Health Organization, 1988); D. A. Henderson, *Smallpox: Death of a Virus,* (Amherst, NY: Prometheus Books, 2009).

limited health resources. Key to the ultimate success of smallpox eradication was India, the most populous of the endemic countries and the one that consistently recorded the largest number of cases and posed some of the most difficult operational problems. The Horn of Africa was the last stronghold of smallpox, a sparsely settled area lacking in resources and a special challenge as the programme struggled to reach completion.

This chapter explores several little known aspects of how the concept of eradication as a practical goal originated, first in veterinary medicine; how it later began to be applied to human disease; and, finally, how the decision was reached to apply it to smallpox. It describes how smallpox eradication was originally agreed upon in the World Health Assembly in 1959, largely as a political gesture. Thereafter, the programme languished for nearly seven years. Even when an "intensified" programme was given new life at the eighteenth World Health Assembly in 1966, many delegates to the Assembly, doubted its chance of success and were concerned that its failure would damage the credibility of the organisation. Expected voluntary contributions were far less than expected, key leaders in the WHO resented a targeted "vertical programme" and unenthusiastically provided needed support. Eventually, even as the goal appeared to be in view, potentially fatal setbacks were narrowly avoided.

The Concept of Eradication

Use of the word, eradication, with respect to a disease did not arise until the latter part of the nineteenth century. Some have mistakenly attributed the concept of smallpox eradication to Jenner, who, in 1800, wrote: "Cow Pox, an antidote that is capable of extirpating from the earth a disease which is every hour devouring its victims."[2] This, of course, was little more than an optimistic hope, not a realistic expectation of a possible accomplishment. Eradication as a practical term for an operational programme was first used in 1884 when, in the United States (US), a veterinary programme

[2] W. R. Le Fanu, *A Bio-Bibliography of Edward Jenner, 1749–1823* (London: Harvey and Blythe, 1951).

was undertaken with the specific objective of eradicating bovine contagious pleuropneumonia from the country. Although due to an organism imported from Europe, it was moderately widespread. Success was achieved within five years and other zoonotic diseases were subsequently tackled in the US and Europe with the objective of achieving area-wide, regional or national interruption of disease transmission. The programmes were referred to as "eradication programmes".

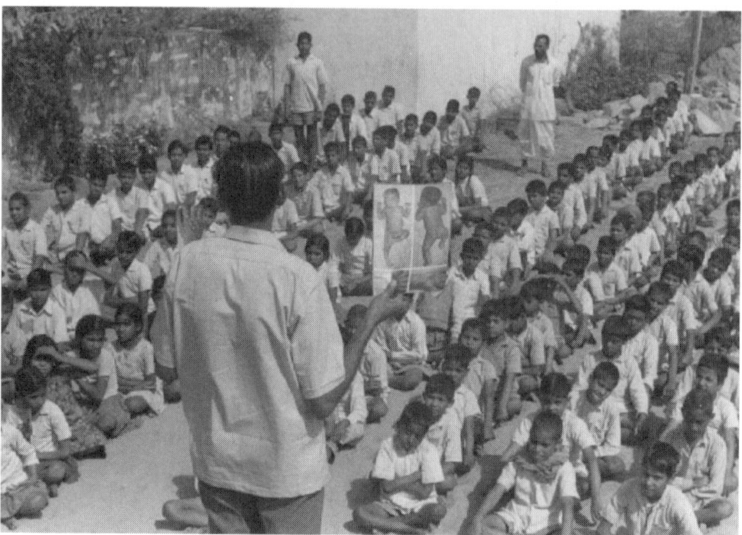

FIGURE 1.1: The search to find smallpox cases. An Indian search worker shows to school children a picture of a smallpox patient and asks if they know of other cases. All reported cases were prominently investigated and village contacts vaccinated to prevent spread of the disease, c. 1973/74.

Source: © World Health Organization.

The possibility of eradicating a human disease was first proposed in 1888 by a leading public health personage of the day, Dr Charles Chapin, Health Officer for the State of Rhode Island. He argued that preventive measures for any disease, if diligently applied, could potentially lead to eradication and, specifically, he cited tuberculosis as a worthy first objective. Nothing came of this proposal.

In the US, public health at the turn of the century was in its infancy, responsibility devolving primarily on towns and cities. There were no national health programmes as such. The idea of undertaking a programme to eradicate a human disease lay dormant until 1909 when, through the philanthropy of John D. Rockefeller, a Sanitary Commission for the Eradication of Hookworm was created and over the following decade, programmes were initiated throughout the southern US and in fifty-two countries on six continents. The strategy called for improving sanitation by the construction of privies and treating children who were found to be infected. No attempt was made to monitor the success of this effort until some thirteen years after it began. At that time, it was discovered that, even where programmes were well conducted, hookworm infections persisted in the community, albeit the infections were somewhat diminished in severity. The programme was abandoned but a precedent was directed for other international eradication efforts.

In 1915, an international yellow fever eradication programme extending throughout the countries of South and Central America was established by an International Health Commission of the Rockefeller Foundation. A programme strategy had evolved from empirical observations which found that yellow fever transmission could be stopped over a wide area by destroying the urban breeding sites of *Aedes aegypti* mosquitoes in towns of more than 50,000 persons. In smaller communities, special programmes were conducted only when outbreaks occurred. Progress was impressive and extensive areas of Latin America became free of yellow fever. However, in 1932, a reservoir of the virus in monkeys was discovered. Eradication of the virus was impossible.

The principal driving force and strategist for the critical stages of the yellow fever eradication programme had been Dr Fred Soper, a brilliant, dominating, demanding and persuasive figure who believed passionately in the concept of eradication. As he visualised the tactics for disease eradication, success lay in "vigorous and effective action".[3] He believed that with a tightly-managed, authoritarian

[3] J. Duffy, ed., *Ventures in World Health: The Memoirs of Fred Lowe Soper* (Washington DC: Pan American Health Organization, 1977).

administrative structure, many diseases could be eradicated. He disdained scientific research and believed that if he could obtain a national commitment to undertake an eradication campaign, available resources and strategy were of secondary concern and these could be worked out as the programme progressed.

In 1947, Soper was elected Director of the Pan American Sanitary Bureau (PASB, now known as the Pan American Health Organization or PAHO) which provided him a platform and forum to pursue eradication on an international scale. At the XXIII Conference of the PASB (1950), and at Soper's insistence, the Directing Council (effectively, ministers of health of the countries of the Americas) approved regional programmes for the eradication of yaws, smallpox and malaria. This was the first instance in which smallpox eradication was decided as a serious objective to be pursued on an international scale. The Bureau had only a miniscule budget and a very small staff but the decision was consonant with Soper's principle of first obtaining a commitment for the task and worrying later about strategy and funding.

Soper had had no prior interest in smallpox control or eradication. His advocacy stemmed from opportunism. In 1947, New York city had experienced an outbreak of nine cases of smallpox resulting from an importation from Mexico. However, fear had reigned and some six million persons were vaccinated. During European visits, Soper learned of a more effective, heat stable smallpox vaccine that had been developed and sought to bring this discovery to the Americas. He believed that such a vaccine would be of special value to the US and would demonstrate the value of the Bureau as an international health agency that could offer something of value even to its biggest contributor.

The Bureau's resources were sufficiently sparse that, for smallpox eradication, it could do little more than provide general encouragement to the countries and technical support to a few national laboratories for vaccine production. Expenditures for smallpox in 1953 amounted to $11,124 and averaged about $40,000 annually thereafter. Nevertheless, the countries themselves took action and, by 1966, all countries except Brazil did become smallpox-free.

A Global Commitment to Smallpox Eradication

In 1953, the first Director-General of the WHO, Dr Brock Chisholm, proposed to the World Health Assembly that a practical world programme, of importance and value to every country, should be undertaken, one that would require concerted international action and would demonstrate "the importance of WHO for every Member State".[4] He took note of the smallpox eradication programme in the Americas and proposed that a global smallpox eradication programme be initiated with a five year budget that provided $131,000 per year. The report was not enthusiastically received. Delegates argued that smallpox was a regional or even local problem and that insufficient knowledge was available to undertake such a programme which "might prove uneconomical and would not . . . add to the prestige of the Organization".[5] The Assembly rejected the proposal and asked that the proposal be further studied—a routine, polite form of rejection.

Until 1958, no further interest in smallpox eradication was evinced at the Assembly. However, that year, Dr Victor Zhdanov, Deputy Minister of Health of the erstwhile USSR (referred to as Soviet Union hereafter), presented a formal lengthy report and proposed a programme of four to five years to eradicate smallpox throughout the world. No mention was made of the then eight-year-old smallpox eradication programme in the Americas. The reason for his initiative, as Zhdanov later explained, stemmed from the frequency with which the Soviet Union had had to deal with imported cases and outbreaks in the Central Asian Republics resulting from importations from other Asian countries. As he reasoned, the Soviet Union, in the 1930s, had interrupted smallpox transmission nationally, including large areas with limited health services, transportation and communication. Thus, it seemed to him that all developing countries should be able to do likewise. To

[4] World Health Organization, "Proposals for World-wide Campaigns: Smallpox", Official Records of the World Health Organization, no. 48, 1953.

[5] World Health Organization, "Proposals for World-wide Campaigns".

facilitate these efforts, the Soviet Union pledged large quantities of vaccine.

For the Soviet Union, this was the first Assembly it had attended after a nine-year absence from the United Nations Organization. In welcoming the return of Soviet participation, the delegates wanted to be responsive to its proposals. Accordingly, they asked Director-General Marcelino Candau to undertake a study of the financial, administrative and technical implications and to report back to the Assembly in 1959.

The Director-General's subsequent report to the Assembly called for little in the way of additional resources. Underlying this was his personal belief, as well as that of a number of delegates, that eradication was impossible. A principal argument was that eradication would require vaccination of all peoples throughout the world. As he pointed out, this was patently impossible as there were, for example, tribes in the Amazon who seldom come out from the jungle. The Director-General's plan called for the endemic countries, some fifty-nine in all, to undertake vaccination programmes using their own or donated resources. The WHO would offer technical assistance when requested and would assist in initiating vaccine production. The plan was accepted and a medical officer was recruited for the WHO headquarters. Over the next six years, WHO staff members were recruited to provide assistance in five of the smallest endemic countries. Total expenditures amounted to about $150,000 per year.

Each year at the Assembly, the Soviet delegates complained bitterly that the WHO was not making adequate resources available for the programme; that, except for vaccine being donated by the Soviet Union, little help was being offered, and that the WHO seemed to be preoccupied with malaria eradication. The fact was that global malaria eradication, begun in 1955, was proving to be far more costly and less effective than had been hoped. The US was contributing heavily to this programme and one-third or more of the regular budget of the WHO was assigned to malaria. The WHO malaria staff numbered 500 to 600, a contrast to the handful working in smallpox eradication.

Other countries joined the Soviet Union in asking the Director-General to provide, in his annual budget, more resources for smallpox eradication. This, however, was a problem because the industrialised countries, the major contributors, objected every year to increases in the Organization's budget, even in amounts sufficient to offset inflation. To provide more resources for smallpox eradication meant cutting budgets for other programmes. The Director-General temporised by arranging for an Expert Committee to be convened in 1964 to consider the situation and to provide advice. Eventually, the committee pointed out that reporting was so poor that it was impossible to offer definitive strategic advice. The committee did recommend that vaccination of as many as 80 per cent of the population might not stop transmission and that, the goal must be to vaccinate 100 per cent of the population. This only served to reconfirm the Director-General's view that eradication was impossible.

At each of the subsequent assemblies, 1964 and 1965, increasing dismay was expressed about the lack of progress in smallpox eradication and the failure of the Director-General to propose larger allocation of funds. Repeated requests were made by the organisation for voluntary contributions to the programme but few responded. Meanwhile, the malaria eradication programme was beginning to founder and was requiring all of the discretionary funds that could be mustered. A significant potential contributor for the smallpox campaign was the United Nations Children's Fund (UNICEF) but it had committed large resources to the malaria programme and its Director bluntly stated in the Assembly that it "would be unable to participate in a world-wide mass eradication campaign against smallpox as it had against malaria".[6]

The World Health Assembly of 1966 marked the final turning point in reaching a decision about smallpox eradication. The Director-General had been instructed to present to the assembly that year a plan and an augmented budget for the programme, utilising funds from the regular budget of the Organization. A small WHO working group, including myself, was convened and a ten-year

[6] Fenner et al., *Smallpox and its Eradication*, 409.

programme plan was drawn up. It called for total expenditure of $180 million for a programme beginning in 1967 and concluding in 1976. The expectation was that 75 per cent of the cost would be borne by the endemic countries themselves with international assistance from the WHO budget and the remaining 25 per cent would come through voluntary donations. For 1967, the Director-General asked for $2.4 million for smallpox eradication. This was 35 per cent of the estimated international assistance requirement for the first year. Voluntary donations of $4.2 million would have to be raised. This was optimistic considering that annual requests for donations during previous years had seldom netted more than $200,000 to $300,000. The Director-General was reasonably confident that confronted with these fiscal realities, the Assembly would decide not to pursue smallpox eradication any more vigorously than it had in the past.

Unexpected Developments in the US

Meanwhile, in November 1965, President Lyndon Johnson unexpectedly announced that the US would provide support for a five-year programme to eradicate smallpox and control measles over a contiguous block of eighteen countries in West and Central Africa. It was anticipated that equipment and teams could be in place in most countries by early 1967. The decision represented the unexpected culmination of events that had begun some six years before.

The chain of events began in 1961 with studies of a new measles vaccine in Upper Volta. They were conducted by staff from the US National Institutes of Health and local health officials. For Africa, the possible availability of a measles vaccine was especially important as the disease was not infrequently fatal in young children. These initial studies demonstrated the vaccine to be fully satisfactory. Subsequently, at the request of the Upper Volta government, the United States Agency for International Development (USAID) supported a national measles vaccination programme for children under six years of age. One year later six West African French-speaking countries successfully petitioned USAID to receive funds to support a four-year programme of measles vaccination in their countries. In 1964, this offer was extended to eleven countries. Help was needed for organising campaigns in each of the countries and USAID turned to the Communicable Disease Center (CDC) for help. I was then Chief of the Surveillance Section which included small units dealing with measles and smallpox vaccination. To part with eleven staff members for six month assignments was impossible.

Moreover, from a public health standpoint, we thought it unwise to initiate a costly measles vaccination programme which the countries could not possibly sustain. Most of the countries then had insufficient resources to buy yellow fever vaccine at less than 10 cents per dose, let alone measles vaccine costing $1.75 per dose.

At the CDC, we developed an alternative proposal which called for a five year programme of smallpox eradication and measles control extending over a contiguous geographic block of countries. This did not solve the problem of sustaining a measles vaccination effort after cessation of the USAID assistance. However, it would at least establish a regional smallpox eradication programme that could be sustained because smallpox vaccine cost only pennies per dose. In addition, this effort would necessarily have to incorporate a contiguous block of countries, some French- and some English speaking because of the large nomadic groups moving across open borders.

The cost of such a programme was estimated to be at least five times greater than USAID had budgeted, primarily because of incorporating populous Nigeria, Ghana and Sierra Leone. As expected, USAID rejected this proposal. However, we had anticipated this would be the opening of discussions as we sought to reach some intermediate alternative that we could manage and USAID could fund. In November 1965, however, much to everyone's surprise, President Johnson decided to support the full eighteen country programme. As it was later learned, the administration had been seeking a possible US initiative that could be announced as a special contribution in support of the UN International Cooperation Year. It was to prove to be a critical impetus to the faltering WHO smallpox eradication commitment.

For the May 1966 World Health Assembly, the subject of intensifying the global eradication effort was scheduled for debate yet once again. The US delegates were instructed to pledge American support for an international programme "to eradicate smallpox completely from the earth within the next decade".[7]

The Decisive Eighteenth World Health Assembly

The WHO budget for 1967 was the focal point of debate. The Director-General's proposed budget without smallpox eradication was $49,115,000, an increase of 12 per cent over the preceding year, largely reflecting inflationary adjustments. If the delegates desired to provide the support that he believed necessary for smallpox eradication, a budget of $51,515,000 would be required, an overall increase of 16 per cent. The debate was a lengthy one with many countries objecting in principle to the proposed substantial increases in budget; many questioned the feasibility of smallpox eradication itself; others expressed doubts about launching a new eradication programme at a time when the flagging malaria eradication campaign needed all the resources that could be mustered. Eventually, the budget was put to the vote. A total of fifty-eight votes were required for approval of the budget incorporating the smallpox eradication effort; sixty votes were cast in favour. The budget was approved by the narrowest margin in the history of the Assembly.

Director-General Candau, believing that the eradication of smallpox was impossible, was most unhappy that the special budget including the programme had been approved. His displeasure was directed particularly at the US whose advocacy for eradication, he believed, had been a deciding factor in the vote. He indicated to the US Surgeon General that he wanted an American to direct the programme so that when the programme failed, the US would be seen to be a principal party at fault. He asked specifically that I be assigned.

Soon after the Assembly, the Surgeon General met with me to inform me that I was being assigned to Geneva. I declined the proposal citing, in particular, my considerable new responsibilities as Director for the recently approved African programme. That programme, as I pointed out, was critical in determining the

[7] D. A. Henderson, personal papers.

feasibility of eradication. If smallpox transmission could be stopped in these African countries, then the world's most heavily infected and with the least resources, global eradication might be possible. Moreover, I shared the view of many that the prospects for global eradication were not bright given the fact that only $2.4 million would be available, less than that being made available by USAID for the West and Central African programme alone. Voluntary contributions amounting to several times the budgeted amount were to be solicited but there had been little response to such solicitations in past years. Finally, there were WHO's well-known problems of developing and operating coherent international programmes what with six very independent WHO regional offices that were unaccustomed to working closely together. The Surgeon General said he had no choice but to order me to assume the directorship of the programme for at least eighteen months in order to get it launched. The assignment was to last eleven years.

When the programme began in 1967, we estimated that there were between ten and fifteen million cases with two million deaths occurring in forty-three countries. Of these, thirty-one countries were eventually determined to have been endemic; twelve countries reported cases resulting from importations. The endemic countries included most countries in Sub-Saharan Africa; the South Asian countries of India, Pakistan (which then included what is now Bangladesh), Afghanistan, Nepal and Indonesia; and Brazil. More than one billion people were living in the endemic countries.

There were some encouraging features, however. Except for Brazil, the Western Hemisphere appeared to be free of smallpox as were countries in North Africa, the Middle East and such Asian countries as Thailand, Burma and Indochina (now Vietnam, Cambodia and Laos). China was also free of smallpox as a result of massive vaccination campaigns in the 1960s, although this was not confirmed until 1979.

Characteristics of Smallpox Favouring Eradication

Smallpox and smallpox vaccine have unique features that taken together made its control and eventual eradication far easier than for any other disease. Most important was that man was the only host and there was no reservoir in nature. The infection itself was of finite duration so that transmission of infection was not possible for more than two to three weeks after onset. Contrary to many medical texts of the 1960s, smallpox did not spread easily or rapidly. The patient transmitted infection only by face-to-face contact and not until he was already sufficiently ill so that he was usually bed-ridden. Following recovery, the patient was immune for life. A single vaccination provided immunity for at least ten years and evidence of a successful vaccination could be readily determined by the presence of a pustule at the vaccination site after seven to ten days or, later, by the presence of a distinctive vaccination scar. The freeze-dried vaccine itself was sufficiently stable so that it could tolerate exposure to 37° Celsius for a month and its application was simple, not requiring a syringe and needle. In areas where *Variola major* had been the prevalent form of smallpox, some 80 per cent of those who recovered had permanent scars, permitting teams to determine both natural immunity and the history of the disease.

The Strategy

The strategy comprised a two-fold approach to be developed simultaneously. First was to diminish the number of susceptibles through vaccination using a freeze-dried vaccine of assured potency, thereby diminishing the extent and rapidity of smallpox spread. Second was to develop a surveillance system requiring weekly reports from all health centres and hospitals. Containment teams (sometimes called "fire-fighting" teams) were to be created to investigate outbreaks and contain them by vaccinating patient contacts and others living in the immediate neighbourhood. The process was referred to as "surveillance-containment". It recognised that smallpox persistence depended on a continuing chain of transmission of virus from case to susceptible contact and by vaccinating patient contacts, the chains of infection could be severed.

An arbitrary goal was established for each programme to assure that 80 per cent of its population was successfully vaccinated.

Quality control teams were deployed to verify this in vaccination campaigns. The quality of the surveillance-containment strategy was measured in terms of the number of days between the beginning of an outbreak and its discovery and the number of days between the report of an outbreak and the date of onset of the last case.

Mistaken Assumptions Necessitating Changes of Strategy and Tactics

In the course of developing the plans for programme operation, four significant assumptions had been made which soon proved to be erroneous and these required important alterations in both strategy and tactics. The four assumptions were

1. That there would be sufficient, high-quality vaccine available to meet the needs of the programme.
2. That a newly developed jet gun, capable of vaccinating as many as 1,000 persons per hour, would play a significant role in increasing the pace of vaccination.
3. That protection provided by primary vaccination was no more than five to seven years and, thus, population-wide programmes involving all age groups would be essential.
4. Rapid progress in containing outbreaks by surveillance-containment would necessitate significant improvements in population immunity.

The First Erroneous Assumption: Vaccine Availability

It was estimated that some 300 million doses of vaccine would be required annually which, if purchased by the WHO at just one cent per dose, would have exceeded the total programme budget. Thus, there was no choice but to plan for all vaccine to be locally produced or donated. This did not, at first, appear to be a serious problem. As of 1967, essentially all countries were vaccinating some proportion of their population against smallpox because the disease was so greatly feared. It was, in fact, the only vaccine then in universal use. Vaccine was produced in seventy-seven different national laboratories, primarily by growth on the flank of a cow, sheep or water buffalo. Taking into account local production, there appeared to be ample vaccine, assuming receipt annually of the pledge of 25 million doses from the Soviet Union and the US supply of all vaccine needed for Western and Central Africa plus possible additional contributions from other industrialised countries.

It was decided, as a first step, to insist that all vaccine for the programme be subjected to independent quality control for potency, purity and stability. The Director-General's office advised that the WHO had no authority to do this. Nevertheless, plans for testing proceeded and laboratories in the Netherlands (Rijks Institute) and Canada (Connaught Laboratories) agreed to perform such tests. Local producers were often reluctantly cooperative and sometimes special pressures were needed to assure compliance.

It was soon apparent that vaccine supply had to be a top priority. In the fifty or so countries that were endemic or bordering endemic areas, not more than 10 per cent of the vaccine then in use met international standards and much of it was in the heat-labile liquid form. In some vaccines, no virus whatsoever could be detected. Meanwhile, it was discovered that most smallpox vaccine laboratories in the industrialised countries had a production capacity of only a few million doses per year and, consequently, few donations could be expected.

Under Dr Isao Arita's leadership, an urgent consultation was convened in Geneva bringing together principal production staff from the UK, Soviet Union, Netherlands, Canada and the US to develop an agreed upon step-by-step production and testing manual. The participants then undertook visits to the larger production laboratories and, using the manual, worked with them to improve vaccine quality. Equipment to permit production of the stable, freeze-dried vaccine was provided by UNICEF. Countries with small laboratories and those with facilities in need of extensive renovation were advised to close down but with the promise that the WHO would supply national needs, primarily using the vaccine of the Soviet Union.

Five years were required to fully solve the problems but, by 1973, all vaccine in use in the programme fully met international standards and more than 80 per cent of it was being produced in the endemic or recently endemic countries.

The Second Erroneous Assumption: Jet Guns Would Revolutionise Mass Vaccination

With large-scale vaccination programmes anticipated, simpler methods for application of the vaccine were sought. The customary vaccination technique at the inception of the programme was to cleanse the vaccination site with alcohol and to let it dry before placing a small drop of vaccine on the skin using some sort of dropper. A lancet was used to scratch through the drop, thus implanting virus in the superficial layers of the skin.

In the US a jet injector gun had been developed in the early 1960s which permitted vaccine under high pressure to be injected intradermally. The vaccine was contained in a 500 dose vial attached to the gun and the gun was powered by a hydraulic pump operated by a foot pedal. As many as 1,000 persons per hour could be vaccinated with more than 95 per cent of the vaccinations being successful. The gun was introduced for use throughout Western and Central Africa and later in some areas of Latin America and Asia. Logistically, however, it proved difficult to assemble sufficient people in one place to permit full use of the gun's potential. Moreover, the guns had a major drawback in that they required daily, skilled maintenance. For every gun in use, there was a need for at least one back-up gun and a mechanic.

Within a few years, however, use of the gun was abandoned because of a simple, ingenious invention, the bifurcated needle, a creation of Dr Benjamin Ruben of Wyeth Laboratories. The needle is two inches long and has a tiny fork at the end. Ruben developed the needle in the early 1960s as a convenient instrument for transferring vaccine from a multi-dose vaccine vial to the skin surface where it could be pressed into the skin using multiple pressures, a method then in common use in the US. When the needle is dipped in the vaccine, a small amount of vaccine adheres to the tines by capillarity, much less being required than when a dropper is used. With the new needle, the usual 0.25 ml vial of vaccine was found to be sufficient to vaccinate 100 persons instead of only twenty-five by customary methods. At the WHO, we developed a new technique for inserting the vaccine—multiple puncture method. The needle was held perpendicular to the skin and fifteen rapid strokes were made. Satisfactory technique could be learned by the average villager with ten to fifteen minutes instruction. Successful vaccinations with this method approached 100 per cent. Moreover, the needles were only US$5 per 1,000 and, with sterilisation, could be reused hundreds of times.

A final step in simplifying the vaccination technique was to abolish cleansing of the skin with an alcohol sponge. Studies showed that normal cleansing of the skin with alcohol did little more than rearrange bacteria. Observations in the field indicated that the very low frequency of secondary infections was no different whether the skin was cleansed or not.

The goals of simplicity and speed were achieved. In the African programmes, vaccinators were able to routinely vaccinate an average of 500 or more persons per day. The only pieces of equipment required were the 100 dose vials of freeze-dried vaccine, a vial of diluent for each vaccine vial, a tube containing bifurcated needles and a pot for boiling and sterilising the needles each night.

The Third Erroneous Assumption: Vaccine Protected for only Five to Seven Years

At the inception of the programme, it was generally believed that revaccination at regular intervals was required to sustain immunity. However, reliable data regarding the duration of protection were not available. Laboratory workers were revaccinated annually; countries required international travellers to be vaccinated every three years; and a number of industrialised countries recommended revaccination every five to ten years. In the endemic countries, however, few persons received more than a single primary vaccination, if they were vaccinated at all. In planning programme operations, it was assumed that to reach a satisfactory level of vaccination immunity, it would be necessary to vaccinate all ages in the population.

However, early surveillance data from Africa and Asia provided puzzling findings. Among adult smallpox patients, in particular, we had expected to see some with a vaccination scar indicating previous successful vaccination but whose immunity had waned. Almost none were found. The explanation for this mystery was discovered by a research team in Pakistan. It found that in households with smallpox, previously vaccinated children had a dramatic increase in smallpox antibodies such as one would expect after a clinical smallpox infection but they showed no symptoms. It was clear that they had experienced sub-clinical smallpox which, like clinical smallpox, provided life-time protection. In endemic areas, many would have been so protected whether or not they were revaccinated.

These findings led to a change in the vaccination strategy to emphasise getting a vaccine scar on every arm rather than endeavouring to vaccinate the entire population.

The Fourth Erroneous Assumption: Smallpox Spread Rapidly and Easily

Classic textbooks emphasised the ease and rapidity of spread of smallpox, likening it to a prairie fire and, thus, we expected to find cases widely dispersed geographically in the endemic countries. These beliefs proved wrong—smallpox did not spread readily like measles and influenza. The long incubation period between infection and onset of illness of ten to twelve days was an important factor.

Only patients with a rash could transmit infection—from the time of onset of the rash until some two weeks later when scabs had formed. Because the rash developed some two to three days after the patient had become very ill and had usually taken to bed, most contact cases were among susceptible household members and visitors. Significant spread did not occur at such as schools or work sites. This made it easier for surveillance teams to trace the spread of smallpox from person to person as it progressed in a continuing chain of infection and so contain outbreaks.

Cases tended to be concentrated in a country rather than being widely dispersed because of the nature of the spread of the disease. This concentration permitted teams to selectively focus their efforts on the most heavily infected areas.

Evolution of the Programme

Because of the paucity of available resources, it was necessary at the beginning to set priorities for the programme. It was decided to utilise WHO funds preferentially in Brazil and Indonesia as these two populous countries did not abut any other endemic countries and, once they had interrupted transmission, it was thought that the available funds could be shifted to other countries in Asia and Africa. Meanwhile, the US had made a commitment to support eradication programmes in eighteen (later twenty) countries of Western and Central Africa, programmes to be directed by CDC and its programme Director, Don Millar. The WHO encouraged the initiation of programmes in other endemic countries but few advisers and only limited additional resources could be made available. The last of the endemic countries, Ethiopia, began its programme in late 1971.

Details regarding each of the country and regional programmes from January 1967 until the occurrence of the last case in October 1977 are set forth in detail in the book, *Smallpox and its Eradication*. A brief summary is here included to offer continuity between the events leading up to eradication and to the critical events that threatened to thwart the achievement of eradication during its concluding years, 1975–77.

Progress during the programme's first six years was dramatic and exceeded expectations. The twenty countries of West and Central Africa interrupted smallpox transmission in 1970, Brazil in 1971 and Indonesia in 1972. By the summer of 1973, the only endemic countries were Ethiopia and four countries of Asia—India, Pakistan, Bangladesh and Nepal. Importations of cases into other countries were diminishing in number and were quickly being controlled.

Despite growing optimism regarding the possibility of achieving eradication by the end of 1976, well within the ten year goal, finances continued to be severely constrained. Voluntary contributions were far less than had been hoped; the Region of the Americas, despite being free of smallpox, refused to permit its allocation of funds to be transferred; and from the WHO, there was a growing disparagement of "vertical" programmes, citing smallpox eradication as an example, as contrasted to "horizontal programmes" (i.e., development of Basic Health Services).

On the positive side, strong support was being provided by CDC in the form of experienced epidemiologists and managers; young volunteers from the US, Austria and Japan were making important contributions in Ethiopia and a growing cadre of dedicated, international staff were dealing ever more effectively with a host of challenges. Their efforts were materially aided by WHO's administrative staff who had overall responsibility for budget, personnel, internal audit, etc., and who went to considerable efforts to provide support to the programme.

By the summer of 1973, India, with its 600 million population, was reporting more than three-fourths of the world's cases. It was recognised to be the ultimate and most problematic challenge to the achievement of eradication. There were armies of vaccinators, albeit performing poorly, and large numbers of Indian supervisory staff but the methods for surveillance and containment that had worked well in other countries, were not interrupting transmission. Some argued that India and the Ganga River Basin must possess unusual ecological characteristics that served to make this area a natural "home" of smallpox, such as was thought to be the case with cholera.

Epidemiological studies, however, revealed that failures to detect outbreaks rapidly and to contain them were primarily responsible. Frequent travel throughout India appeared to be an important factor. India was served by a surprisingly extensive rail and bus system which was inexpensive and heavily used. Religious festivals drawing hundreds of thousands were common; commuter traffic was heavy in urban areas; and it was discovered that entire families often travelled from urban areas to their home villages when one of the family members became ill.

It was decided that more rapid case detection and containment was needed. Thus, in the summer of 1973, it was decided to utilise a proportion of the veritable army of public health staff to search for smallpox in every village in India over a seven to ten day period and to take immediate measures to contain the outbreaks that were found. The first searches began in October of that year utilising some

120,000 health workers. The completeness of the initial searches left much to be desired but tens of thousands of unreported cases were found, many times more than anyone had expected. The sudden surge of reported cases alarmed WHO staff, as well as high levels of the government, and served to generate a substantial increase in political support for the programme. The searches were repeated every two to three months thereafter, with a focus on the areas with continuing transmission. Containment measures were made increasingly stringent. As performance improved, the objective was altered to that of contacting every house in India during the search.

Little more than eighteen months after the special programme began, the last outbreaks were discovered and contained. Meanwhile, Pakistan and Nepal, adopting similar methods, became free of smallpox and by May 1975, smallpox in Asia was confined to limited areas in neighbouring Bangladesh. There, it was the beginning of the summer season, a time when smallpox spreads slowly and can reasonably readily be contained.

Meanwhile, in Africa, programmes had progressed well and by May 1975, smallpox was restricted to limited areas of just one country, Ethiopia.

Concluding Chapters: On the Brink of Defeat

In May 1975, the global eradication of smallpox appeared to be all but a certainty and perhaps achievable within a year. In Bangladesh, experienced WHO and national staffs were working well. By August, there were less than twenty infected villages (i.e., those that had experienced a case within the preceding six weeks) and effective national searches were being conducted utilising some 24,000 health staff. Ethiopia appeared to be in a less favourable situation; civil war had broken out the year before but Ethiopian and national advisers continued working actively although at considerable personal risk. With smallpox limited to only two countries substantially more resources could be made available as well as experienced staff from other countries. For Ethiopia, contributions of two helicopters, as well as a fixed-wing aircraft, eased the difficult transport problems and neighbouring countries assisted by undertaking surveillance and containment measures near their borders but within Ethiopia.

Beginning in August 1975, however, two major problems arose that seriously threatened the possible achievement of eradication.

Bangladesh

In August, the Director-General and I were scheduled to travel to Dhaka to meet Bangladesh national leaders to encourage them and their staff in the apparent final phase of the eradication of *Variola major*. We had been in India to celebrate its annual Independence Day and, Prime Minister Indira Gandhi's proclamation of India's freedom from smallpox for the first time in its recorded history.

En route to the airport after the ceremonies, we were informed that Sheikh Mujibur Rahman, the first President of Bangladesh and revered father of the newly independent country, had been assassinated along with his family in a military coup. All flights were cancelled; the borders were sealed; all communications were suspended; and Indian troops began mobilising to deal with what was expected to be a mass exodus of refugees. We knew from experience that civil war and refugees were a certain prelude to rapidly spreading epidemic smallpox.

The veteran national and international staff had endured four difficult years contending with smallpox during major floods, civil unrest, and famine and were well accustomed to adversity. Wisely, they dispersed all their vehicles from a motor pool to rural areas so as to preclude their being seized by military or rebels. They suspended most operations for some two weeks but gradually resumed activities. Surprisingly, the country remained relatively calm and on 16 October, a three-year-old girl, Rahima Banu, developed smallpox, the last case in Asia and the last case of *Variola major*, the severe form of the disease.

Ethiopia

Smallpox eradication in Ethiopia was an especially daunting task. It was the last infected country and the challenges were awesome. The population of 25 million was widely dispersed in small villages across a vast highland area and in nomadic groups that roamed across the Danakil and Ogaden Desert crossing unmarked borders into Somalia and Djibouti. It was said that half the population lived more than three days walk away from any accessible road. The health infrastructure was at an early stage of development and there were few professional staff.

The programme did not start until late 1971, almost five years after the global smallpox programme had been decided. Until then national and international malaria programme staff had persuaded the Minister of Health of the need to focus all efforts on malaria eradication which was heavily supported by bilateral funds. The malaria programme was the dominant health programme with a staff of some 8,000 workers, more than twice the number of all other health staff personnel. Reluctantly, the government agreed to a smallpox eradication effort and provided twenty-one Ethiopian sanitarians to assist. Gradually, the international staff grew with the US, Japanese and Austrian Peace Corps-type volunteers being added and, later, additional WHO staff but the numbers of national and international staff were not large and much of the transport was on foot and by mule.

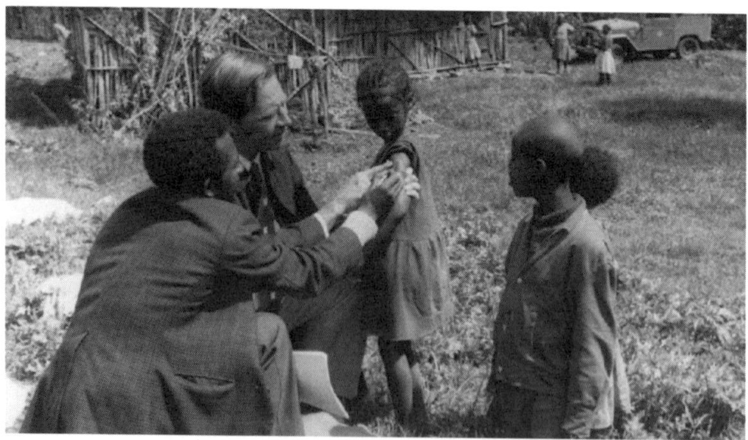

FIGURE 1.2: D. A. Henderson with Ethiopian health officers checking to see that the child has been successfully vaccinated, c. 1974/75.

Source: © World Health Organization.

In addition to the many logistical problems, security problems became increasingly serious late in 1974 as a major revolution occurred, the Emperor was deposed and a new government undertook a number of radical changes. Pockets of armed rebellion emerged throughout the country, open warfare began with neighbouring Somalia, and Eritrea declared itself independent. The problems persisted throughout 1975 and 1976; the volunteers were withdrawn; and international staff, except for those in the smallpox programme, were not permitted to venture outside of the capital. An intrepid group of Ethiopians and international staff continued work despite all but impossible obstacles. Finally, in June 1976, they detected an outbreak in a small village in the Ogaden Desert. They contained the outbreak and searched everywhere for other cases. To their surprise, they found none.

Seven weeks elapsed and celebrations were cautiously being planned in hopes of being able to celebrate the global eradication of smallpox. These were rudely interrupted by a report from neighbouring Somalia of five cases in Mogadishu, the capital. Immediate consultation by the WHO staff confirmed that the cases were indeed smallpox but where, specifically, they had been infected could not be ascertained. Somalia had been conducting a special surveillance and vaccination programme since 1969 and reported that eighty-five per cent of its population was vaccinated. Between 1972 and 1975, the country reported only 38 cases, all importations from Ethiopia.

The WHO epidemiologists worked with Somali staff to search suspected areas in Mogadishu but the government would not permit them to travel outside of the city. Through December 1976, thirty-four cases were officially admitted to the Mogadishu hospital and containment measures were taken for these cases. However, the staff were suspicious that the government might be suppressing reports but the magnitude of this deception was only realised some two years later when confidential records were discovered showing that more than 500 patients had actually been admitted to the hospital in Mogadishu but were sequestered in a special section of the building.

Not until March 1977 did the government agree for the staff to travel outside of Mogadishu and for the assignment of additional WHO staff to cope with a steadily increasing number of cases with apparent sources of infection in other parts of Somalia. Through June, the staff grew steadily, eventually comprising some forty WHO and Somali epidemiologists and more than 2,500 Somali surveillance agents. Many of the cases were among the nomads but simply finding these roving nomads in the high brush of the vast desert areas was a real challenge. A disturbing discovery was the fact that continuing chains of infection were possible in groups as small as thirty-five to fifty-five people and for up to five months. The number of cases reached a peak of 1,388 in June. There were some 3,229 cases in all before transmission was stopped.

On 26 October 1977, twelve months after the first alert that smallpox was present in Somalia, the last case was diagnosed and containment measures taken. As problematic as this last epidemic was, a concurrent threat was that the disease might be carried to Mecca at the time of the annual pilgrimage and from there spread to pilgrims coming from all parts of the world. In Ethiopia and Somalia, the milder variola minor had been prevalent and, even when ill, patients could move about reasonably readily. With Somalia being so near to Mecca, there are, every year, tens of thousands of Somalis who make the overland trek to the holy city. To forestall problems, special vaccinators were assigned to pilgrimage groups to assure that all were vaccinated, to vaccinate others who might later join the group and to report possible cases. None occurred.

A Legacy of the Smallpox Eradication Programme

During the evolution of the smallpox eradication programme, two important developments were fostered that are serving to help transform the practice of public health in much of the developing world. One was to build on the experience and methodology of the smallpox vaccination programme to incorporate the use of other vaccines. The second was to begin to utilise a surveillance network for the purposes of planning and monitoring other vaccine preventable disease efforts.

Early in the smallpox eradication programme, it became clear that an effective large-scale vaccination effort could be implemented utilising surprisingly small number of vaccinators and attaining good coverage of the population. By deploying vaccinators in teams, close supervision was possible to assure proper vaccination technique and preservation of the vaccine. Quality control was possible by revisiting a sample of the villages seven to ten days later to assure that coverage was at least 80 per cent and that more than 90 per cent of the vaccinations had been successful.

It seemed only logical to consider expanding the efforts of the smallpox vaccination teams to administer a number of vaccines. By the mid-1970s few developing countries were utilising diphtheria-pertussis-tetanus (DPT) vaccine or poliovaccine and none outside of the West and Central African programme used measles vaccine. To further discuss the possibilities for a more extensive vaccination effort, an international meeting of senior health staff from a number of countries was convened in 1970 at the PAHO headquarters in Washington. From this came the recommendation to the World Health Assembly that it approve an "Expanded Programme on Immunisation" which, for the developing countries would include six antigens (smallpox, diphtheria, pertussis, tetanus, measles and polio). In 1974, this was approved by the World Health Assembly.

At the inception of that programme, it was estimated that less than ten per cent of children in the developing world were receiving DPT, polio or measles vaccines. Gradually, the new initiative gained momentum, finally meeting its target of reaching 80 per cent of children throughout the developing world by 1990. In the course of the programme, the polio eradication programme emerged.

In the developing world, the concept of surveillance as an active instrument for programme implementation and monitoring was effectively unknown. The surveillance system that was established for smallpox was an innovation for most countries but it was able to be more readily established than had been expected. It was critical for our understanding of the epidemiological behaviour of the disease, for prioritising programme operations and for monitoring progress. It involved receiving each week a report from every health centre and hospital regarding the number of cases of smallpox as well as basic data on each patient (age, sex, village, date of onset, vaccination status). Data were analysed concurrently at each administrative level and by the WHO programme staff in Geneva.

Such reports are now being gathered on poliomyelitis and, in the Americas and some other countries, for cases of measles and rubella. Other diseases are being added to the list.

The Future of Eradication

In 1980, only months after smallpox was declared to have been eradicated, the first of many conferences was convened to explore what next should be eradicated. Many different diseases have been proposed and considered at the different meetings but only two eventually have been agreed upon by the World Health Assembly—poliomyelitis and guinea worm disease. Programmes for each of these diseases have now been in progress for more than twenty years. Their expected target dates for eradication passed many years ago. They each continue to face formidable obstacles as prospects for eradication stretch into a distant and uncertain future.

My views regarding the feasibility of other public health eradication programmes were tempered in the fires of smallpox eradication. It never occurred to me to contemplate the possibility of another disease being eradicated, at least for the foreseeable future and I do not recall such an initiative ever having been discussed among our senior staff. However, only months after the World Health Assembly declared that smallpox had been eradicated, all manner of enthusiasts emerged to advocate for adoption of other global eradication targets such as polio, measles, urban rabies, hunger, road accidents and many more.

For those of us who had lived the smallpox eradication experience, who knew the sacrifices that were necessary and who knew how narrowly it had succeeded, it was difficult to understand how anyone could take the proposals seriously. In 1982, at a meeting of the American Philosophical Society I stated:

> Many have proposed that another disease should be targeted for eradication and another global campaign launched. In my opinion, there is no other disease which possesses so many characteristics favourable to

> an eradication effort or for which we now have available, effective, simple and inexpensive measures for prevention or treatment. Although smallpox eradication may now seem to have been comparatively straightforward, I recall well innumerable instances in which the programme balanced on a knife edge between success and disaster, decided by such events as an unexpected change in government, a cessation of hostilities or a heroic exhibition of dedication, courage and leadership by WHO and national staff. There were a multitude of miraculous and timely events. . . . Even with these, eradication just barely succeeded.[8]

I suggested that, for now, the most appropriate goal was to eradicate the word "eradication" as applied to a global programme. I have seen nothing since 1982 that would warrant altering that conclusion.

[8] D. A. Henderson, "The Deliberate Extinction of a Species", *Proceedings of the American Philosophical Society* 126, 1982, 461–71.

2

A Miracle Happened There: The West and Central African Smallpox Eradication Programme and its Impact

Joel G. Breman

Introduction

This chapter draws upon personal perspectives of the West and Central African Smallpox Eradication Programme in twenty African countries between 1966 and 1971.[1] In fact, it was a Smallpox Eradication/Measles Control Programme. The Africans were really more interested in measles control than in smallpox eradication, but that is not the focus of this chapter.

I worked for thirteen years on smallpox. I lived in Guinea from 1967 to 1969 as a medical epidemiologist, also covering Senegal. From 1972 to 1976, I was responsible for smallpox and other disease surveillance in eight West African francophone countries belonging to the Organisation de Coordination et de Coopération pour la lutte contre les Grandes Endémies (OCCGE), a regional public health and research organisation, based in Bobo-Dioulasso, Burkina Faso. From 1977 to 1980, I was at the Smallpox Eradication Unit, World Health Organization (WHO), Geneva, completing and confirming eradication. During the end of the global programme, I was responsible for

[1] Benin (Dahomey), Burkina Faso (Upper Volta), Cameroon, Central African Republic, Chad, Equatorial Guinea, Gabon, Gambia, Ghana, Guinea, Ivory Coast, Liberia, Mali, Mauritania, Niger, Nigeria, Republic of the Congo, Senegal, Sierra Leone, Togo.

Map 2.1: West and Central African Smallpox Eradication/Measles Control Programme, 1966–71

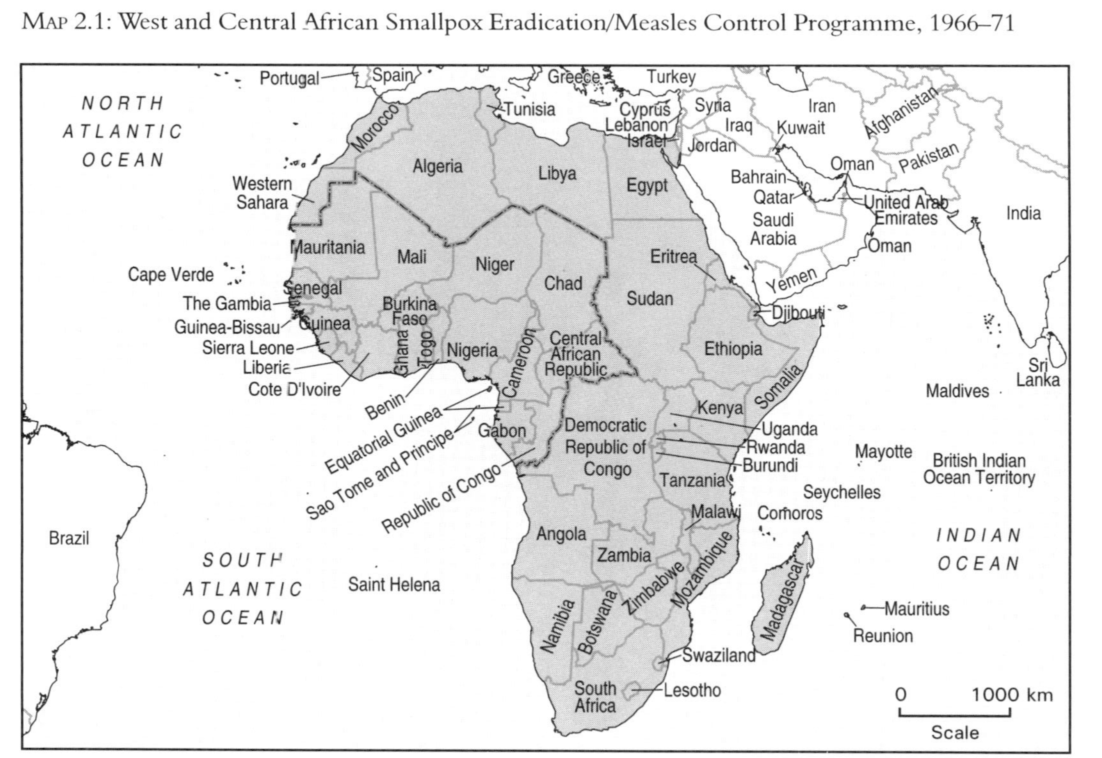

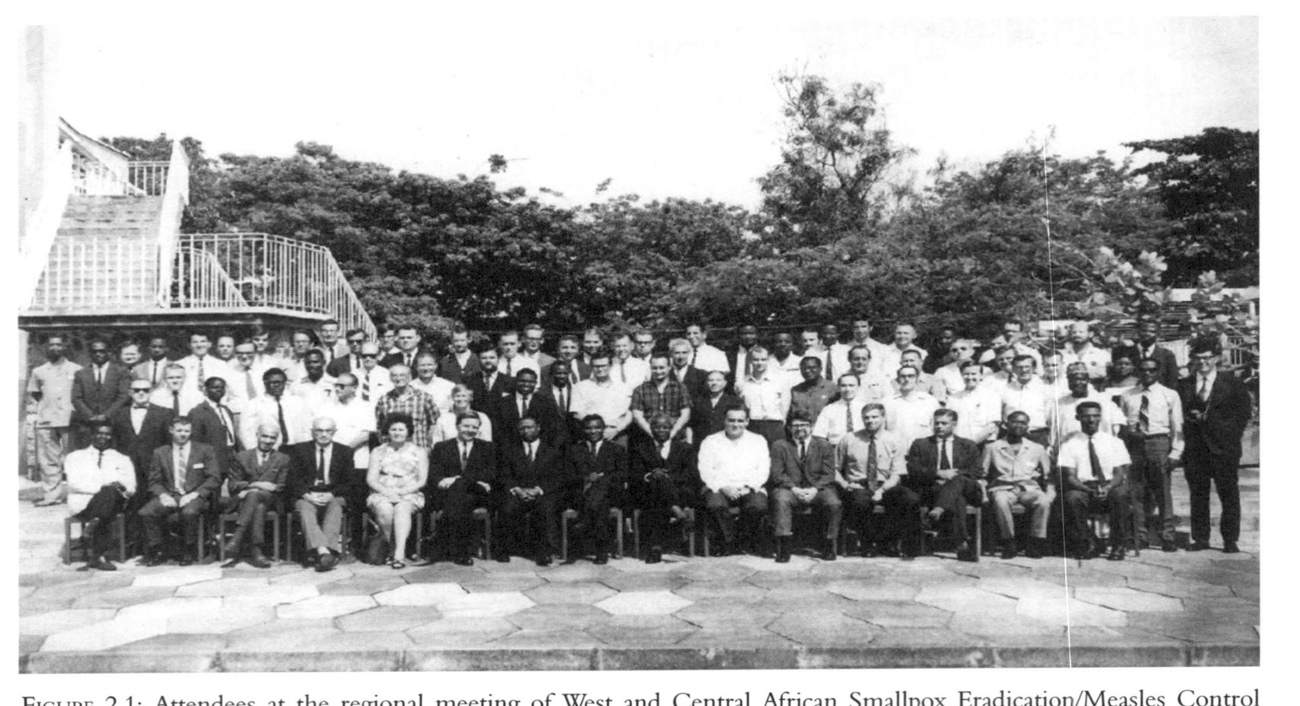

FIGURE 2.1: Attendees at the regional meeting of West and Central African Smallpox Eradication/Measles Control Programme, Lagos, Nigeria, 1969. Names listed below.

First row, L to R: Dr N'Dow (Gambia), Mr Eddins (CDC), Dr Shafa (WHO), Dr Meiklejohn (WHO), Dr Marennikova (Soviet Union), Dr D. A. Henderson (WHO), Dr Cheick Sow (OCCGE), Dr Smith (Nigeria), Dr Ademola (Nigeria), Dr Labusquière (OCEAC), Dr Millar (CDC), Dr Foege (CDC), Dr Nugent (WHO), Dr Prince-Agbojan (Togo), Dr Grant (Ghana)

Second row, L to R: Mr Rothstein (CDC/Nigeria), Mr Wade (CDC/Nigeria), Mr Aliyu (Nigeria), Mr Davis (CDC), Dr Glockpor (Togo), Dr Mayer (WHO), Mr Thornton (CDC/Sierra Leone), Dr Curtis (USAID), Mr Charter (CDC/Chad-Guinea), Miss Jones (CDC/Nigeria), Mr Olson (CDC/Liberia), Dr Mebitaghan (Nigeria), Dr Barry (Guinea), Mr Jenkins (CDC/Nigeria), Mr Newberry (CDC/Ghana), Mr Donoho (CDC/ Nigeria), Dr Tchelle (Niger), Dr Roots (CDC/Niger), Mr Okoh (Nigeria), Dr Imperato (CDC/Mali), Dr Binson (Ivory Coast), Dr Lane (CDC), Dr Durand (CAR), Dr Poirier (Cameroon), Mr McEnaney (CDC/Nigeria), Mr Robbins (CDC), Dr Ruben (CDC), Mr Ewen (CDC/CAR), Mr Adepoju (Nigeria), unknown, Mr Evans (CDC/Nigeria), Dr Breman (CDC/Guinea)

Third Row, L to R: unknown, Dr Cummings (Sierra Leone), Mr Hicks (CDC), Dr Hopkins (CDC/Sierra Leone), Mr Masso (CDC/Niger), Mr Copland (WHO), Mr Leonard (CDC/Mauritania-Senegal), Dr Melchinger (CDC/Ghana), Dr D'Amanda (CDC/Burkina Faso), Dr Arnold (CDC/Nigeria), unknown, Dr Pifer (CDC/Nigeria), Mr Griggs (CDC), Mr Agle (CDC/Togo), Mr West (CDC/Nigeria), Dr Thompson (CDC/Nigeria), Mr Malberg (CDC/Guinea), Dr R. Henderson (CDC/Nigeria), Dr Foster (CDC/Nigeria), Mr Flanders (CDC), Mr Bond (CDC), Dr Adetosoye (Nigeria), Dr Yekpe (Benin), Mr Helmholz (CDC/Senegal), Mr Omolola (Nigeria), Mr Friedman (CDC/Mali), Dr Sentilhes (Burkina Faso), Mr Issoufi (Niger), Dr Roux (Chad), Mr Lapointe (CDC/Chad/Guinea), Mr Godfrey (CDC/Ivory Coast), Dr E. Coffi (Ivory Coast).

Source: Photograph provided by the author.

poxvirus research, focusing mainly on human monkeypox, and certification of global eradication. In all these postings overseas, I was a United States Centers for Disease Control and Prevention (CDC), then the National Communicable Disease Center, staff member.

I will focus on my experiences in Guinea to reflect what happened elsewhere in the programme, while granting the great diversity of history, cultures, politics and disease ecology in the areas where we worked. I know I am representing over fifty CDC West and Central African pox-fighters and more than a thousand African and expatriate health workers, and all their families—to whom I dedicate this chapter, but exempt them from any errors.

What is a miracle? The Merriam-Webster dictionary defines a miracle as "an extraordinary event manifesting divine intervention in human affairs." Certainly, eliminating a disease in less than five years that had been firmly established in West Africa for over a millennium was miraculous. The "divine power" was the fortuitous convergence of modern science and technology; the political will of newly emancipated African countries committed to a better life for their people, including smallpox eradication; devoted African health workers; a US presidential decision to support the WHO and the African programme through the United States Agency for International Development (USAID); and a group of young, naive, brash, irreverent, idealistic, and adventurous medical and operational staff from the CDC.

The Background

The history of smallpox shows how long and deeply imbedded this disease had been in Africa. Smallpox in West and Central Sub-Saharan Africa is a story of at least 1,300 years of continuous disease with 34,000 unbroken chains of human-to-human spread. The disease probably came to Western Africa by camel from Egypt in the seventh century A.D. with the penetration of Islam into the western and southern parts of the continent. Over the next several hundred years there were periodic internal wars within and between the great and small African empires and then exploration and colonisation,

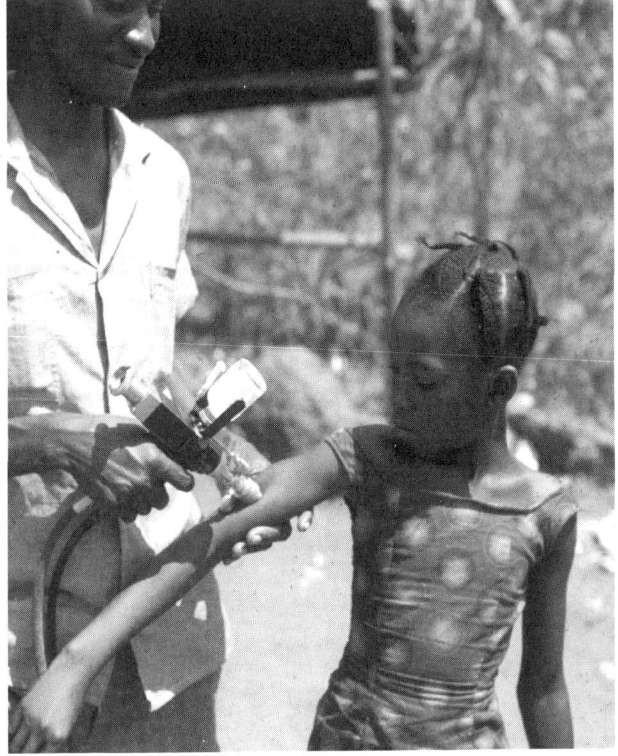

FIGURE 2.2: Guinean nurse giving smallpox vaccination using the Ped-O-Jet injector.

Source: Photograph provided by the author.

starting with the Portuguese in the sixteenth century followed over the next three centuries by the Belgians, British, French, Spanish, Germans and Dutch. In addition, slave trading carried smallpox along its routes within Africa, to Europe and the Americas. Disease flourishes when communities are disrupted by war and oppression. The miracle of vaccination began late in the eighteenth century with Edward Jenner's discovery, but it was only in the early twentieth century that a form of dried vaccine developed by Lucien Camus in France was sent to Guinea and the Ivory Coast.

During the early-to mid-twentieth century the great mobile health teams of the French military, initiated first by Eugene Jamot in the Cameroon to combat sleeping sickness, showed that diseases could be confronted in a rural environment, if not defeated. Smallpox vaccinations, using liquid vaccine prepared on the flanks of cows, became a mainstay of some of these mobile health team activities. These early vaccines were heat labile and had miserable potency. While many persons were vaccinated, relatively few were ever immunised, mainly in the capitals, and with minimal impact on the disease. Successful smallpox immunisation 'take rates' (representing vesicle development and scarring on the skin at the vaccination site) reported from the Belgian Congo ranged from 9 to 64 per cent, averaging 38 per cent in the 1930s and 1940s. From 1935 to 1944, 26 million vaccinations were given in French West Africa to a population that was 16 million in 1944. Yet smallpox raged. Epidemiological approaches to smallpox control were not generally used. Fearing the visible wrath of smallpox, and having a notion that the disease could be passed between humans, villagers often constructed isolated huts for patients. Traditional healers were consulted and they thrived because little else was available.

Between 1957 and 1965 all of the West and Central African countries in the programme had gained independence; the exception was Liberia which became independent in 1847 and was a refuge for slaves from the US. Freedom allows a young country the audacity to build on others' experience, to try new things and to make mistakes. Freedom brings idealism and a shared passion to a mission; focused passion gets things done. African communal reliance expressed as "pan-African nationalism"—practiced for a while in Guinea and a few like-minded countries—created the milieu to make the eradication miracle come true more easily. Regrettably, independence and nationalism by themselves do not alleviate poverty.

Atlanta

I first arrived in Atlanta and then Guinea forty years ago with my wife Vicki from a residency in internal medicine. I had essentially no foreign experience. My French was fragmentary. Fortunately, my medical training was at the School of Medicine, University of Southern California and the Los Angeles County General Hospital, the largest hospital in the US where we saw mainly indigent patients, many with complex pathology. The outstanding paediatrics and communicable diseases departments were headed by Paul Wehrle of the University of Southern California, an alumnus of the CDC, who recruited me. We were trained in Atlanta in epidemiology and biostatistics in the Epidemic Intelligence Service course; the virologic, clinical, epidemiological and control features of smallpox and measles; and in vaccinology and vaccines. We learned about tropical diseases, African history, culture, anthropology, geography and weather patterns. In 1967, B. B. Waddy from the London School of Hygiene and Tropical Medicine came and spoke on the British experiences dealing with the great scourges. One pearl from Waddy that I never forgot was that the entire economic system of West Africa depends upon people getting paid promptly at the end of the month. Those going to francophone countries studied French for a couple of hours at night after the other courses.

The two month training covered basic repair and maintenance of vehicles, refrigerators and vaccination equipment. We learned all about the Ped-O-Jet vaccine injector, a hydraulic, foot-pedal-armed portable inoculation gun. The CDC teams were trained in the summers of 1966 and 1967 and left in fits and starts, depending on how successfully negotiations were concluded with countries, USAID missions, embassies, in some instances the WHO, the OCCGE in Bobo-Dioulasso, Burkina Faso (formerly Upper Volta), and the Organisation de Coordination pour la lutte contre les Endémies en Afrique Centrale (OCEAC), another francophone health organisation based in Yaoundé, Cameroon. The lightning-illuminated nights in Atlanta in the summer of 1967 were exceedingly hot and humid, a good preparation for life in Africa.

I was amazed at how young and bright the Smallpox Eradication Programme's leaders were in Atlanta. Don Millar, aged 33, was the Director. He was a jovial, brilliant epidemiologist with a syrupy Virginian accent, wry humour, and skilled in playing guitar, and singing folk and bluegrass anthems. Millar had just returned from training at the London School. Young Bill Foege, also a CDC alum and guitarist, was a medical missionary working in eastern Nigeria when the civil (Biafran) war erupted in mid-1967. Foege returned to the CDC as a regional smallpox programme supervisor and became an important strategist, rising in later years to become the Director.

D. A. Henderson had worked on organising the West and Central African programme in the mid-1960s and getting President Lyndon Johnson's office to support the endeavour fully. His epidemiological skills, including doing landmark studies on influenza, polio and other diseases, led to his becoming a protégé of Alexander Langmuir, the famed founder of the CDC Epidemic Intelligence Service. D. A. Henderson was also in his 30s when he went to Geneva in 1966 to head the global Smallpox Eradication Programme. Indeed, most of us who worked in the CDC Smallpox Eradication Programme were in our 20s and 30s. A special comment is needed about the public health advisors, called operations officers. One of the CDC's main innovations was developing and assigning talented administrators and managers to health programmes. They managed the crucial organisational, logistics, transport, equipment and budgetary domains. Having operations officers in Africa was the brainchild of Billy Griggs and Bill Watson, top CDC managers. All operations officers were trained in epidemiology and many used these skills well. Several operations officers rose to important positions at the CDC, WHO, Red Cross, the Carter Center and elsewhere. Among the many greats, Bob Helmholz in Senegal went on to become Chief Administrative Officer of the Onchoceriasis Control Programme in West Africa and the Chief Administrator of the South East Asian Regional Office of the WHO. Jean Roy, former Peace Corps volunteer, directed smallpox eradication in Benin (formerly Dahomey), child survival programmes in the Democratic Republic of Congo (formerly Zaire), and initiated an innovative combined malaria and measles control programme while at the International Federation of Red Cross and Red Crescent Societies in Geneva.

Guinea Reflections

My time in Guinea could be divided into three overlapping emotional periods—frustration, isolation and jubilation. Guinea is slightly larger than the United Kingdom. In 1969, the country had about 3.75 million people speaking three major local languages, representing the Susu, Peuhl and Malinké populations, with French as the national language. The life expectancy of a Guinean newborn in the 1960s was twenty-nine years. The mid-century birth rate of 62 per 1000 and infant mortality of 216 per 1000 live births were among the highest in the world. The economy was in shambles, the French having left abruptly when the Sekou Touré-led nation voted not to remain with the French community of nations after independence in 1960. Infrastructure was fragmentary—the only major paved road went out to Kindia, about 150 km east from the capital, Conakry, and there were few road-worthy vehicles. There was one doctor per 160,000 persons in rural areas, where over 90 per cent of the people lived. Most Guinean doctors were called "médecins Africans", a pejorative term used by many expatriates for a high level physician's assistant who received special training, usually in Dakar. Very little medical equipment was present and drugs were always in short supply. Who else was in Guinea when I arrived? The communists and socialists. Few Western countries wanted to offend the French so the Soviets, Czechs, Yugoslavs, North Koreans, mainland Chinese and Cubans came. The Chinese and Cubans were in several regions throughout the country and, while the iron curtain was still down, we often met and occasionally dined together at a regional governor's house. I took special satisfaction when the foreigners were ordered to be vaccinated by regional authorities. After one long trip, I found that the infectious diseases and smallpox isolation ward at the main hospital in Conakry had been turned into an acupuncture unit run by the "red" Chinese. Fortunately, by then smallpox was in full retreat.

Early, my bureaucratic masters at the CDC were aggravating, insensitive and unresponsive. They immediately began demanding reports on accomplishments, projected programme activities and budgets even though we had barely arrived. Shipments of vaccines, refrigerators and other materials did not arrive when scheduled or arrived without prior notification. The worst, by far, was not receiving the vehicles, the legs of the programme, until the second year of field activities. On top of this, the Guineans initially appeared indifferent and suspicious of us—neo-colonialists from the West.

One reason the Guinea programme began in 1967, rather than 1966, was the absolute need to get a written agreement for me, Don Malberg and later Russ Charter, the operations officers, to travel anywhere in the country unimpeded. No other foreigner had this special laissez-passer. Henry Gelfand of the CDC gets the credit for this negotiating coup. Henry and George Lythcott, who headed the programme's regional office in Lagos, pounded out these crucial agreements country-by-country and with other partners, including those at USAID in Washington DC. Henry and George and others involved deserve special battle ribbons for this unheralded task.

While we used the US embassy telecommunication system, other means of communication were miserable. I received one telephone call from Atlanta in almost two years and had to go to the main post office to get it. The few phones in the country were unreliable and I never had one. Mail often took months, particularly for my medical journals which came by ship every three months—if the ships were allowed to dock in the Conakry harbour. Transport in the field was by foot, vehicle, boat and the Russian Antonov or Ilyushin airplanes. These planes were used by Air Guinée and noted for their abrupt take offs and descents and thick fog and ice producing air conditioning systems. Messengers were the usual mode of contact. Throughout the entire time I was in Guinea, I was anxious—worried if the equipment and vehicles would arrive in time, if the team members would be vaccinating according to schedule, if the roads would be open and passable and, most concerning, if smallpox was becoming uprooted. I was also anxious about the well-being of Vicki, who was not yet used to my long periods away without communication. In time, she accommodated, worked at the US embassy as a nurse, and travelled with me. And, she too fell in love with the kind and welcoming Guineans and with Africa.

Guinea had the second highest rate of smallpox in the world in 1967, after Sierra Leone directly to the south. Most smallpox patients in Guinea were detected in areas bordering Sierra Leone which had widespread disease. We tried to coordinate our vaccination efforts with Don Hopkins and Jim Thornton of the CDC, and E.

C. Cummings, the national Sierra Leonean programme Director, based in Freetown. After a two week training period, starting in late 1967 during Ramadan, we began moving east along the Guinean southern endemic border beginning in the region of Forécariah. Our goal was 80 per cent coverage, based on the dictum, incorrect in my experience, that this level of "herd immunity" would stifle epidemics and eliminate disease. Indeed, reliance on mass vaccination, forwarded initially by the WHO and the CDC as the major tactic was discarded within one year of my arrival. Mass vaccination continued, but was superceded by the "eradication escalation" strategy based on disease epidemiology and containment. This strategy was presented by Bill Foege at our regional programme meeting in June 1968 in Abidjan. He has credited the idea to a Royal Commission on Vaccination of 1896. Using seasonal occurrence of outbreaks to direct control efforts made immediate sense to me and others. As smallpox was a dry season disease, the fewest outbreaks and cases occurred during the heaviest summer rains. Working smart, not only hard was a good mantra for any task—even though it was clear that we would be slogging through the mud.

The Guinean health workers were the most dedicated, hard-working, self-sacrificing, field-wise and innovative group I have encountered. The hard-earned agreements with USAID mandated that African governments were responsible for all salaries and lodging of their staff, even in the field. This was a mistake. Because of the absolute poverty of the government and the Ministry of Health, there was no field allotment of any type. The teams slept and ate in the villages where they were working. Their meagre salaries were delivered to them or their families erratically. Bangoura Alécaut, my counterpart, Chef, Service National des Grandes Endémies (Chief of the Preventive Medicine Services), made the decision to have all-male teams stay in the field virtually without a break the entire vaccination year, from December 1967 through June 1968, and after the heavy rains, from September 1968 through June 1969. He said that they would not come back to work if given time off between regions. He was right, but several personal problems surfaced: marital separation and divorce; delinquency among school-age children; and impotence upon returning home were just a few of the laments. Yet, the team members loved the adventure. They had the rare opportunity to see their beautiful country and meet and serve their people. They also understood the treacherous toll that smallpox and measles had taken on Guineans and were proud that they were doing something about it. The teams were invariably welcomed warmly in the villages, often with singing, dancing and patriotic manifestations. These benefits muted the hardship.

I am not sure the Guineans were expecting the organisational surprises that I urged and that came early. First, despite not having many roadworthy vehicles nor a large contingent of "volunteer" nurse workers, we immediately took one vehicle and driver for the independent evaluation team. One of our best and most respected vaccination team leaders, Kourouma Famba, an "agent technique de la santé", a highly skilled chief nurse, was trained in cluster sampling survey methods to determine smallpox and measles vaccine coverage. Shortly after the vaccination teams passed through a region and city, Famba's team visited a representative number of villages and people, asking who had and had not been vaccinated by age and sex; he looked at arms to read primary and secondary vaccination reactions, and recorded 'take rates' to assure smallpox vaccine potency and good technique. Concurrent, statistically valid programme evaluations and close supervision were not traditions in African health programmes. Second, because of lack of transport we combined the Field Supervisor's role with that of an advance information team. Joseph Kourouma, a demanding leader, was superb at solving field problems; he met regional and local authorities and publicised when and where the vaccination teams would be arriving in each village or assembly point with written notice of date, time, place and exactly what would be done. He also arranged the teams' regional reception and lodging. Using the well-organised Guinean political and administrative machinery assured outstanding cooperation throughout the country. Third, six months after the programme began, we designated another team with a vehicle for the crucial smallpox detection and containment activities headed by Sékou Bangoura. When extra transport was available we could perform mop-up vaccinations in villages and towns with low coverage;

for this we often left vaccine and instructions for regional health workers.

I mentioned that we did not have vehicles when we began. The US embassy donated a few road unworthy Willy-Wagoneers and older trucks from a previous measles vaccination campaign. The Guineans came up with a Russian dump truck and a Land Rover. Our car park and maintenance areas were the UNICEF "garage", a sparsely supplied lot with several auto and truck carcasses used for spare parts, and the US embassy motor pool. We were truly a shaggy-looking army when we started. Gasoline was not easy to find and we sometimes purchased this from the black market, what Guineans called "le marché americain". We did not have much motor oil either, and had to go to Sierra Leone to buy it. The only blistering argument I had with Dr Alécaut was when I saw one of our vehicles rolling down the street in a parade, filled with young political revolutionaries during one of the hastily called national holidays. About the same time, another programme vehicle was being used by Alécaut personally. When I insisted on regaining the needed transport at our private confrontation, Alécaut blasted me very sternly. "Monsieur le Docteur – personne dans le programme n'est indispensable" (No one here is indispensable), meaning I could leave if I did not like the way things were done. For a while, I thought I might be kicked out of Guinea as yet another counter-revolutionary. Within a few weeks both vehicles were returned to the programme. Bangoura Alécaut became a lifelong friend.

The wisest comment about transport in Africa came from Pierre Ziegler, a legendary Frenchman who had spent sixteen years as Chef des Grandes Endémies in Chad. Ziegler was later chief of the WHO smallpox programme in the Democratic Republic of Congo and first Director of the West African Onchocerciasis Control Programme. He wrote, for every vehicle in the field you should have one in reserve along with an ample supply of spare parts. This could be applied to refrigerators, vaccine cold boxes, and Ped-O-Jet injectors. For many years, while based in Burkina Faso, I carried spare axles and two spare tyres in my one weary Land Rover.

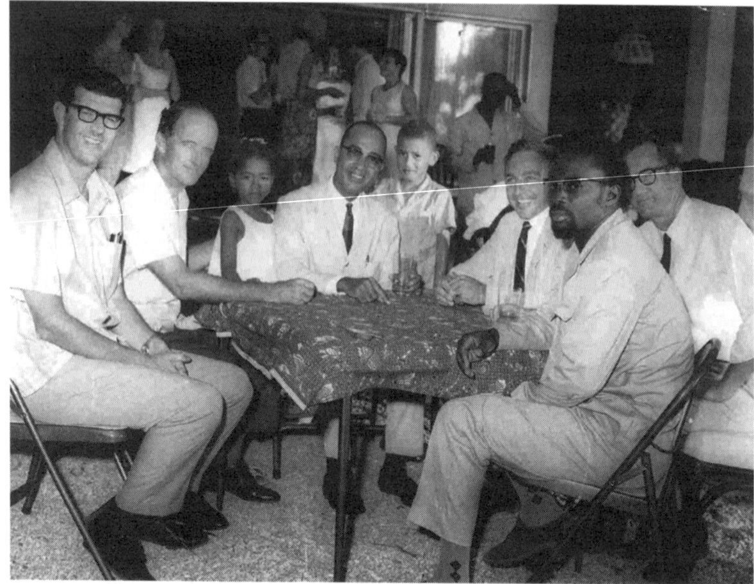

FIGURE 2.3: Reception for the Smallpox-Measles Programme, Conakry, Guinea, 1969.

FROM L TO R: Dr Joel Breman (CDC), US Ambassador Robinson McIlvaine, Dr Bangoura Alécaut (with Therese and Andre Alécaut), Mr Don Malberg (CDC), Mr Joseph Kourouma, Mr Al Ford (USAID).

Source: Photograph provided by the author.

"Truth Be Told", Guinean Worries

I never felt confident that smallpox was gone from Guinea until shortly before I left in June 1969. Outbreaks were reported in multiple regions before we vaccinated, during vaccination and, most discouragingly, after we vaccinated and had investigated and contained outbreaks. The outbreak areas were among the most difficult to reach. Faranah region, the birthplace of the President, had smallpox in several villages near international markets along the Sierra Leone border. Local health authorities there flat-out fabricated mop-up vaccination records after low coverage during the initial campaign. Another large outbreak surfaced in a very difficult to reach isolated Atlantic island off the coast of Kamsar, Boké, where there was a large bauxite deposit. And, in Forécariah, in southwest Guinea, there were multiple importations from Sierra Leone. Some of these importations started smoldering outbreaks despite vaccination coverage of close to 90 per cent. Over 210,000 vaccinations were given over 14 months in this one region having a censused population of 95,000; measured coverage was over 90 per cent with 98 per cent 'take rates'. Nevertheless, by late December 1968, one year after we began field work, the onset of illness in the last smallpox patient began in Forécariah. Regrettably, the investigation was delayed to early January 1969 so the record shows that Guinea still had smallpox in 1969. Were we smallpox-free?

In April or May of 1969, after four or five months of no cases, I was given a telegram late in the afternoon from the Ministry of Health stating that smallpox was present in Mamou city, 300 km from Conakry. Arriving with a team that night we went immediately to the house of the Director of Public Health. I showed him the telegram. He said yes, he had sent the telegram to Conakry; yes there had been smallpox in the hospital when he sent the cable; yes, the month and day were the same . . . but the telegram had been sent one year earlier! It had remained buried on someone's desk in the health ministry. I was still unconvinced even though the Director verified the old date on the cable, so we all went to the hospital. By lantern we saw a patient with severe but typical chickenpox and took specimens. After viewing every patient in the hospital and reviewing outpatient and inpatient record books for the past year, I was convinced. There was no smallpox in Mamou. Two months later I left Guinea as scheduled, in jubilation.

Programme Pearls

What did we learn in Guinea, clinically and epidemiologically? Smallpox was easy to diagnose during an epidemic, often difficult at other times. I saw the spectrum of disease, from patients with the fulminant, flat, lethal form to those with a few lesions. Severe chickenpox and allergic reactions were diagnostic conundrums, particularly when the patient appeared to be the only case.

The disease affected smaller communities and was not explosive. While smallpox was horrific, feared and disfiguring, it affected relatively few people in rural communities and spread slowly. Close, face-to-face contact with an infected patient was virtually always needed for transmission.

Surveillance and response were the major keys to eradication. I am convinced that identifying outbreaks promptly, first during the low transmission season in 1968 and later at any time, was the reason we had such rapid success. Smallpox, then suspected smallpox, became a public health emergency in everyone's eyes. With this attitude and responsive action, smallpox melted.

Once outbreaks were reported or found, we investigated them compulsively. Our contact tracing covered places and persons that cases had visited within three weeks before and three weeks after they became ill. This assured that we knew all possible sources of disease acquisition and dissemination. These places and persons were investigated and vaccinated. If they were in neighbouring regions or countries the authorities were notified. Repeat visits to outbreaks identified more patients and assured complete containment. Sometimes patients were kept hidden because of severe illness or shame so house-to-house searches were necessary.

We collected specimens. Again, severe chickenpox can resemble smallpox. Monkeypox, seen in later years in West and Central African countries, looks exactly like smallpox clinically and does not spread avidly between humans. You never know for sure until the laboratory confirms the diagnosis. A table showing the number of specimens collected in formerly endemic areas with negative smallpox virus results, and listing the alternate diagnoses, is the best ending for a report on eradication. Sceptics—and there are many during the eradication programmes—will accept laboratory results more than other explanations.

One key to success was using good freeze-dried stable vaccine. 'Cold was gold'. Creation and maintenance of the cold chain was especially challenging, particularly in Upper Guinea where the temperature could go well over 40° Celsius and electricity was practically absent. The portable kerosene-powered refrigerators were essential as were ice chests packed with 'chiens froids' ('cold dogs'), and thermoses for field use. Measles vaccine was especially fragile and teams were urged to open the ten or fifty dose vials when they had a suitable number of persons to vaccinate.

'Herd immunity' is an oversold concept and not applicable unless you have a fully isolated herd. This is never the case in Africa. Susceptible populations are constantly arriving; the birth rate is high, and 5 to 10 per cent of the resident population is always on the move—we gave about 5 per cent of all vaccinations at 'barrages sanitaires' or road blocks—and waves of in- and out-migration can be predicted or occur unexpectedly.

The operational lessons I took from Guinea

Disease eradication is best approached as a military campaign. This requires understanding the enemy, bold assaults, micro-planning, meticulous logistical support and divining the changing environment. Above all, clarity of objectives and a feasible and flexible operational plan need to be shared openly with staff and all partners involved in the programme. Everyone needs to know what is expected of them and how to do it.

Mobile teams and direct village contact are essential for disease eradication. While village assembly points were sometimes used, these were never more than 5 km from any village. If we would have used the sparse health units exclusively the programme would have failed.

Keep your promises. For this, you will earn respect, devotion from your co-workers and a superior performance. Show up when you said you would. Pay the workers when you said you would. Deliver the vehicles when you said you would. Underpromising and complete follow-through leads to overachieving.

Train, train and retrain. Workers at every level want to improve their skills. If you cannot do it properly yourself, the field workers will not do it properly. This applies to giving a vaccination, doing an investigation, repairing a Ped-O-Jet injector or maintaining a vehicle.

Sleep in the field with the teams. Nothing raises the morale of your troops more than sharing the hardships and joys of the battle. One's presence shows the community that you are interested in them and their culture. You will see and learn more about diseases and their environment from overnight or extended village visits than by returning home each night or from perfunctory visits to a capital city. You will also save gasoline.

Communicate to those doing the work in the field frequently and frankly. Field workers are the heroes of eradication. Programme workers at every level are motivated more by professional satisfaction—seeing how they are doing compared to other teams, other districts, other regions, other countries—than by anything else. Everyone wants to be the first to eliminate a disease. No one wants to be last. A brief, illustrated surveillance bulletin is a great motivator. Name names. In Guinea we had one such bulletin; Sierra Leone called theirs *The Eradicator*.

Don't ask, don't tell. Just before the second year of operations a group of unfamiliar faces appeared in our brief retraining session. Dr Alécaut asked if we could afford to give them some vaccine for "northwest Guinea". The answer was yes, of course. Only later did I find that they were with the liberation movement in Guinea Bissau, a country that won their independence from Portugal in 1973. I was once asked by a 'diplomat' to record all military movements I observed within the country and report them to him. My answer was no: our surveillance was very different from his surveillance. Any action that would compromise the programme was forbidden.

The West and Central African Programme

Expanding my thoughts to the West and Central African programme, I have several observations. What was learned? Most importantly, the salient experiences and lessons from 1966 to 1971 were adapted successfully to the remaining smallpox endemic countries after 1971 by tens of thousands of national and global staff.

Smallpox could be eliminated from a very large region without 80 per cent coverage. The programme area was about the size of the continental

US and had 120 million persons in the late 1960s. Nigeria had well over half of the population and the eleventh highest incidence of smallpox in the world in 1967; we could have used more field staff in this country. The "escalation eradication" strategy, later called "surveillance containment", concentrating on rings of priority contacts, works.

Develop, test and use new technologies. The Ped-O-Jet injector was costly and hard to maintain for some countries, but it really worked in West Africa after being tested successfully by the CDC in Tonga and Brazil in the early 1960s. In Guinea, each vaccination team gave about 2,000 smallpox vaccinations per workday over two years. The bifurcated needle was not used in the West and Central African programmes early, but replaced all other vaccination devices throughout the world by the early 1970s because of its simplicity and need for only a drop of vaccine.

Dispel myths. Smallpox was not an explosive disease anywhere; it spread slowly taking relatively few victims in its wake. Work by Tom Mack and others in Pakistan in the mid-1960s, by David Thompson and Bill Foege in the famous Abakaliki, Nigeria, outbreak, and others in several countries proved this important point. Traditional healers, while influential, did not impede vaccination in Togo, Benin and Western Nigeria where native medicine and 'fetisheurs' reigned. The smallpox god Shopona in Nigeria was defeated rather than appeased. Several of us from the programme were able to obtain copies of Shopona at our regional meeting in Lagos in 1969, thanks to Ralph "Rafe" Henderson who was the regional office epidemiologist and interested in cultural beliefs about vaccination.

Research is critical for all public health programmes. Descriptive epidemiology defined disease patterns—population vulnerabilities, locations, age and periods of transmission. Laboratory differentiation of the orthopoxviruses (smallpox, vaccinia and monkeypox), and of herpes-varicella virus (chickenpox) was critical. Jim Nakano, John Noble and members of the great CDC laboratory team were essential for confirming the diagnoses and assuring that eradication was achieved. John Obijeski and Joe Esposito of the CDC made major contributions to understanding poxvirus genetics and evolution.

A global poxvirus laboratory network focusing on diagnosis and research in support of the eradication programme was established by the WHO. Nakano, Chief of the WHO Poxvirus Collaborating Center, along with Svetlana Marennikova, Chief of the Moscow WHO Poxvirus Collaborating Center, were leaders in this important endeavour—particularly as monkeypox raised its head in the early 1970s from several West and Central African countries, most notably the Democratic Republic of Congo. Tens of thousands of specimens were tested by the CDC and Moscow laboratories during global certification activities throughout the 1970s and during the 1980s when monkeypox research and surveillance continued.

Be prepared to lose a few battles. Learn from adversity. Who from the programme could have foretold or altered the course of the Nigerian civil war, from 1967 to 1970? Perhaps, someone could have predicted that CDC and WHO efforts to establish high quality, high volume smallpox vaccine production factories in Yaba, Nigeria and Kindia, Guinea, would not succeed because of problems with egg supplies, sterile water, electricity, refrigeration and anything that required moving parts. Yet, it was important to transfer technology and improvise locally. While we were required to use US-made Dodge trucks, they were vastly inferior to the Land Rover and other brands. In later years the Toyota Land Cruiser equalled the Land Rover in reliability and these vehicles could be obtained with managerial creativity.

Listen, listen and listen. Observe carefully. Understand and adapt to local ways. Pascal "Pat" Imperato of the CDC, Ousmane Sow, and colleagues working in Mali documented potentially dangerous, but ineffective variolation practices, how best to deliver health services to nomads and the important role of markets as vaccination sites. Don Hopkins, E. C. Cummings and colleagues in Sierra Leone described the importance of funerals for spreading disease, with contamination occurring during ceremonial washing of the corpse by bereaved family members.

Transfer and adapt what you learn to other countries and organisations and learn from them. Each country improved on what had been done earlier. People get things done but organisations have cachet, networks and resources. The CDC leadership was fully committed to smallpox eradication. David Sencer assigned staff to countries, WHO, OCCGE, OCEAC and other agencies until the job was finished. In late 1976, I was asked by Bill Foege and David Sencer to join the Smallpox Eradication Unit at the WHO when D. A. Henderson left. When I reminded David Sencer that he had urged me to take a domestic post if I wanted to stay with the CDC, he instantly replied that he considered Geneva a domestic assignment.

Without strong leadership the mission will fail. What do we expect in leaders? One who is clear in communicating the mission, objectives, strategies and tactics; has good judgement; is honest and forthright; is receptive to contrarian views; has creativity in introducing ideas; is adept in choosing good lieutenants and delegating authority and responsibility; promotes allegiance to and from field staff and provides incentives. A great leader manages by objective and by example. My view of a successful management scheme is an inverted pyramid with the troops on top supported by a hierarchy of leaders. The finest leader I have known is D. A. Henderson, who, in addition to having the above-mentioned qualities, responded to every letter he received from field staff within forty-eight hours and to longer documents including manuscripts usually within two weeks; he also understood the importance of logistical support. David Sencer, former Director of the CDC, managed by walking around the campus and into offices and laboratories to stimulate and encourage staff; Sencer sent his very best people for extended periods into the field to battle smallpox including his deputy, Bill Watson, the chief administrative officer, who served in India. Bangoura Alécaut inspired respect by insisting on the maximum work performance from each team member. He had great national pride, but knew and compensated for the shortfalls in Guinea. He knew what local, national and international partners could and could not do, and assured that everyone was a winner. All three leaders were decisive, accessible around the clock, chose the right people for the right job and knew how to get money by hook or crook.

In addition, good leaders know the importance of hospitality, social mixing, inclusiveness and humour to gain trust and allegiance. In sum, a leader must tell the story clearly, be devoted and responsive to field staff, have knowledge of the task, good judgement, make good appointments, and be resourceful and shameless in attracting resources. D. A. Henderson has said that every good idea used to eradicate smallpox came from the field, not from headquarters. There never were more than four to six smallpox unit medical or administrative officers at the WHO headquarters, even when thousands of searchers were combing endemic areas. Most of the time the WHO headquarters staff were in the field. In the late 1970s, our smallpox headquarters staff ate C-rations in the WHO dining room to commiserate with the field teams in Somalia to whom we sent these pre-packaged meals.

Impact

The success of the West and Central African programme was a great impetus for success in the rest of the world. If countries with the toughest field conditions, the fewest resources, and the highest disease incidences could succeed, hotbeds of disease in countries in the Indian subcontinent and eastern and central Africa could conquer smallpox and prove that they had done it. Over the next four years, from 1971 to 1975, David Sencer assigned over 250 of his staff for periods from three months to several years to work in smallpox-endemic countries. They worked with national and international colleagues to eradicate the disease and to confirm eradication during the difficult documentation and certification phase which lasted to 1980. The CDC poxfighters usually were WHO consultants and worked as international civil servants. They joined an international fraternity of co-workers with high esprit from dozens of countries. They succeeded in bringing modern knowledge of epidemiology, surveillance, containment, ring vaccination, communications, logistics, teamwork and good management to Afghanistan, Bangladesh, Nepal, India, Ethiopia and Somalia, and to the WHO offices in Geneva and New Delhi. In the field, their allegiance was always to the goal in the countries and organisations where they were assigned. Every major innovation that was discovered or rediscovered in West and Central Africa was used elsewhere, refined locally, tested, improved and transferred again. At the same time, colleagues from other countries were developing innovative approaches with the WHO for detecting, reporting and containing smallpox outbreaks; these included the smallpox and monkeypox identification pictures, house-by-house searches, procedures for dealing with variolation, highly publicised rewards for case reporting and surveillance of massive population gatherings such as those coming to Saudi Arabia during the Haj.

West and Central African countries were not forgotten. The CDC staff joined francophone regional health organisations in Burkina Faso (OCCGE) and Cameroon (OCEAC) to strengthen surveillance and do research in vaccine-preventable diseases, cholera and monkeypox. In 1972, I started my work on malaria in Bobo-Dioulasso, Burkina Faso, at the Centre Muraz, OCCGE. In the early 1970s, Neal Ewen, who had been the operations officer in the Central African Republic's smallpox/measles programme, began a CDC-Burkina Faso collaborative rural disease and demographic project working with the Peace Corps. Tom Leonard, an operations officer who had smallpox eradication experience in Mauritania and Burkina Faso, and Donald Moore, who had been an epidemiologist in Niger, participated in nutritional assessments in the Sahel during the devastating West African drought of 1973.

Inspired by success with smallpox eradication, the WHO began the Expanded Programme on Immunisation about 1975, and its early Director was Rafe Henderson, who later became an Assistant Director-General. He was widely known for refining the vaccination coverage scheme developed by Robert Serfling and Ida Sherman of the CDC and adapting it to Africa. This popular coverage survey approach remains in use. Many others from the CDC have had major influences in global public health. Among these are: Don Hopkins, now at the Carter Center, Atlanta, who is the father of the Guinea Worm Eradication Programme—a debilitating parasitic disease poised to be the second one eradicated. Pat Imperato became the Commissioner for Health of New York City and chairman of the Department of Preventive Medicine and Community Health, State University of New York, Brooklyn. Pat is a renowned authority on West African art and culture. Stanley Foster, professor at the Rollins School of Public Health, Emory University, was the CDC-assigned leader of the Nigerian and Bangladesh smallpox programmes, and worked among smallpox-infected nomads in Somalia. He had done important facial pock mark surveys showing that only 1–5 per cent of smallpox patients were reported to health authorities before the global campaign. Foster and Andrew 'Andy' Agle were architects of a major African child survival programme in the 1980s and 1990s, managed and implemented by the CDC and financed by USAID. Agle had fought smallpox in Togo as an operations officer, and in Afghanistan and Bangladesh. Bill Foege became an influential adviser on global health to President Jimmy Carter and to Bill and Melinda Gates and their foundation.

Many Africans who worked on the programme rose to positions of prominence, usually in preventive medicine and in their ministries of health. Bangoura Alécaut, my Guinean counterpart, became ambassador to the Republic of Congo, Brazzaville, and other Central African countries. One of the youngest nurses in the Guinean programme, Sidimé Banian, graduated from the new medical school in Conakry almost two decades after I first met him.

Perhaps, the most important contributions of the eradication programme are two intangibles—pride and credibility. The pride resides in tens of thousands of health workers for achieving what many thought impossible. Smallpox eradication has given increased credibility to those health workers, their countries, and to national and international organisations participating in the programme. It also changed the minds of those lacking confidence in international cooperation and the United Nations agencies.

While smallpox eradication is a miraculous achievement, I am one who believes the good old days are yet to come. This chapter is based on a presentation given at the Wellcome Trust Centre for the History of Medicine at UCL on 25 April 2007. That was African Malaria Day, now known as World Malaria Day and I wore my malaria tie to remind us of the need to conquer this great African and global peril. In conclusion, my prediction is that the miracle of malaria eradication and that of other great scourges will someday be described from this stage.

I thank David Sencer for encouraging me to tell this story and my adventurous and lovingly supportive wife Vicki and children, Matthew and Johanna, for living it with me.

3

The Eradication of Smallpox from India

Larry Brilliant and
Corrie White Conrad

> Smallpox was always present, filling the churchyard with corpses, tormenting with constant fear all whom it had not yet stricken, leaving on those whose lives it spared the hideous traces of its power, turning the babe into a changeling at which the mother shuddered, and making the eyes and cheeks of the betrothed maiden objects of horror to the lover.[1]

Introduction

As the Second World War drew to a close, and more than a century after the historian Lord Macaulay penned this description of the "always present" smallpox, two-thirds of all countries in the world still had "the pox." Even in countries that appeared free of the disease for a year or a decade, wave after wave of killer smallpox was considered an inevitable, even normal, part of life. But a decade later, in 1959, the world community, through the World Health Assembly, overcame helpless resignation that smallpox was inevitable and undefeatable, and gathered the political will to pass an audacious Russian resolution, committing all nations to work together to conquer this ancient scourge. By 1969, mass vaccination programmes sometimes coupled with quarantine measures,

The authors thank Girija E. Brilliant, PhD for kindly editing this chapter.

[1] T. B. Macaulay, *The History of England from the Accession of James II* (London: J. M. Dent and Sons, 1800).

brought the number of infected countries down to 63. By 1970, smallpox had been beaten down to only 18 countries and by 1974, epidemiologists cheered as the number of endemic countries was reduced to five. But just as eradication seemed tantalisingly within reach and despite huge numbers of people having been vaccinated, smallpox seemed to explode from its ancient homeland of India.

Smallpox was especially tenacious and virulent throughout the sub-continent where *Variola major* killed one in every three people who contracted it. The elimination of smallpox in India was a crucial step towards global eradication and it is often cited as one of the great victories in the history of public health. The diversity of peoples, languages, religions and geographies combined with tense geo-political realities, high population density and a very mobile population made India the world's principal endemic focus for smallpox for many years.[2] India was the historic heartland of smallpox, and the disease played a unique role in commerce and culture—so much so that in the late nineteenth century parliament had passed the tough Bengal Immunity Act requiring compulsory immunisation for smallpox and jail for anyone who refused to be vaccinated. It was a remarkable piece of public health legislation.

In 1973 the World Health Organization (WHO) reported that 60 per cent of the reported smallpox in the world came from India. By 1974 WHO announced that 90 per cent of smallpox cases in the world were limited to four Indian states: Uttar Pradesh, Bihar, West Bengal and Madhya Pradesh. The population of India that year was just under 600 million, divided amongst 21 linguistic states, strong administratively distinct governing units. Health was a "state subject", each state determining its own health priorities. To many planners in the states, and some at the national level, smallpox was not at all the primary health problem. Smallpox accounted for only 0.15 per cent of India's total deaths in 1973 while TB accounted for approximately 5 per cent of deaths that same year and tetanus about 10 per cent.[3] But smallpox was WHO and the world's priority and

[2] Larry Brilliant, *The Management of Smallpox Eradication in India* (Ann Arbor, MI: University of Michigan Press, 1985), 1.

[3] Brilliant, *Management of Smallpox Eradication in India*, 31.

somehow these conflicting priorities between global and national needs would need to be resolved in order for *Variola major* to meet its end on the Indian sub-continent.

This chapter recounts highlights from the story of smallpox elimination in India. Beginning with the history of the National Smallpox Eradication Programme (NSEP) the narrative moves through three defining moments, breakthroughs in "hard science" and field epidemiology merged with superb management and unprecedented public health zeal, culminating with "Zeropox"—a double entendre signally both "zero cases" of the disease as well as the "virus" of contagious enthusiasm felt by smallpox workers that smallpox could be eradicated. The dream of eradicating this ancient disease was a magnet drawing some of the most talented health workers to the Indian sub-continent from dozens of countries, like the highest mountain draws the most adventurous mountain climbers. Smallpox eradication could accomplish a challenging "first" and it attracted a very entrepreneurial leadership and team. Vignettes from their stories—-of people who made smallpox eradication a reality in India—are also included here. But it is very important to remember that only a tiny per cent of leaders of the Indian smallpox campaign were from outside of the country. The international team in India, headed by Nicole Grasset and Bill Foege and including Zdeno Jezek, Lev Khodakevich, Nick Ward and many other wonderful epidemiologists, was outstanding. But it was the Indian doctors and health workers who sacrificed the most. I was privileged to work with some genuine Indian heroes; I think fondly of M. I. D. Sharma, Mahendra Dutta, R. N. Basu, Mahendra Singh, R. R. Arora, C. K. Rao, A. G. Acharia and Zafar Hussain as well as Health Minister Karan Singh and J. R. D. Tata and Sujit Gupta from Tata's and so many others. These are but a few of the tens of thousands of Indian heroes who eradicated smallpox and inspired us all.

History of the National Smallpox Eradication Programme (NSEP)

The Indian effort to conquer smallpox was begun as a completely national activity, but it soon garnered early international support because of the historic importance of smallpox in the sub-continent. In May of 1958, the Indian Ministry of Health appointed an expert committee under the auspices of the Indian Council of Medical Research (ICMR) "to examine the problem of smallpox and to suggest means for its eradication."[4] One year later, Dr V. N. Zhdanov, a Soviet health official, introduced a resolution urging WHO to launch a global campaign to eradicate smallpox in 1959. Increased international attention was focused on India, and combined with a major domestic epidemic in India (168,216 recorded cases and 45,838 deaths in 1958) that catalysed Indian creation of this expert committee.[5] In June 1959, the expert committee recommended that the NSEP be set up to vaccinate the entire Indian population within a period of three years.[6] WHO and the Government of India agreed on a joint commitment to eradicate smallpox in India through NSEP. It took a little over a year to launch pilot vaccination projects in one district in each of the 21 states and in Delhi. By March of 1961 only half of the 23 million people living in the pilot project areas were vaccinated, but the idea of NSEP and a goal of mass vaccination of the entire population was firmly in place.

The Ministry of Health accepted the recommendations of the expert committee and the Smallpox Pilot Project Committee in October 1961, and decided to include NSEP as part of the Third Five Year Plan. The Ministry sanctioned Rs 68,900,000 (approximately $8,600,000) to launch NSEP and in addition to the available funds, the USSR made an initial contribution of 250 million doses of freeze-dried vaccine. The first installment of donated vaccine arrived in February 1962, and a further donation of 200 million doses arrived in 1964.[7] The provision of freeze-dried vaccine was a vital improvement. Previously, vaccine was available only in a liquid form and it was not heat stable. It was not until 1971 that liquid vaccine was effectively abolished in India in favour of the freeze-

[4] R. N. Basu, Z. Jezek and N. A. Ward, *The Eradication of Smallpox from India* (New Delhi: World Health Organization, 1979), 21.

[5] Brilliant, *Management of Smallpox Eradication in India*, 6–7.

[6] Basu, Jezek and Ward, *Eradication of Smallpox from India*, 21.

[7] Ibid., 21–23.

dried vaccine. In addition to the USSR contribution, the United States Agency for International Development (USAID) provided Rs 10,000,000 (about $1,200,000) to aid in payment of salaries and other expenses.[8]

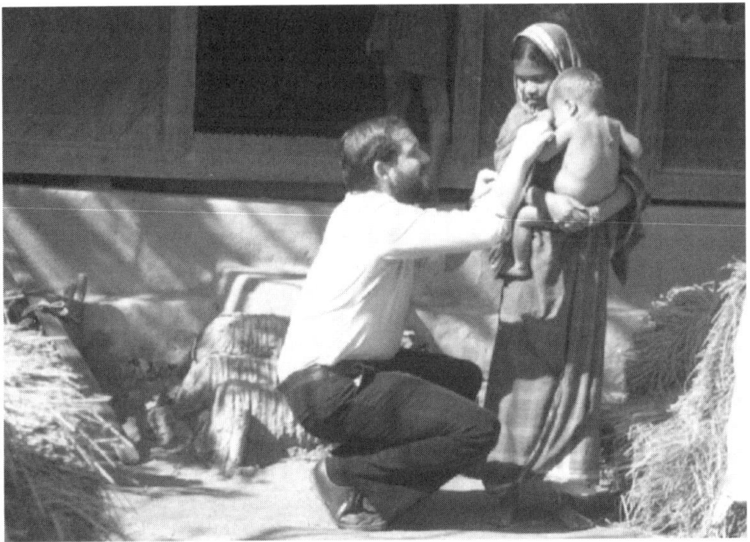

Figure 3.1: Dr Larry Brilliant examines one of the last smallpox cases in India, 1975.

Source: Photograph by Nedd Willard, provided by the author.

In 1962, the first year that India recorded national vaccination statistics, over 32 million Indians were vaccinated; in 1963 the number more than quadrupled to almost 139 million. Often, however, the liquid vaccine, which was still in use, was ineffective. Despite the encouraging vaccination statistics, reported smallpox incidence in 1963 soared to 83,438 cases with 26,360 deaths—more than double the incidence at the start of the NSEP in 1963.[9] India alone accounted for over 80 per cent of all known cases in the world that year, and the case fatality rate was the highest at 31.6 per cent.

[8] Brilliant, *Management of Smallpox Eradication in India*, 9.

[9] Ibid.

NSEP was a three-phase programme: preparation, attack and maintenance. The preparation phase occurred through the pilot projects. During the attack phase the goal was to attain 80 per cent vaccination coverage of the population in 2 years. This goal was in line with the WHO-promoted strategy of mass vaccination at that time, and would have required 351 million vaccinations for India's 1961 population of 439 million people. Based on a study conducted in Madras that showed that most neonatal vaccinations resulted in positive take rates and low complications, NSEP emphasised the importance of vaccinating newborns, but no distinction was made between primary vaccinations and revaccinations in the reporting, so it was not possible to track when someone's first vaccination occurred. [10]

The concept of 'herd immunity' dominated the thinking of smallpox eradicators at that time and had led to the mass vaccination campaigns. It was thought that if enough people in a community were vaccinated and therefore immune to smallpox, the disease could not propagate through the 'herd' of people in that community. WHO and many national governments stressed high vaccination coverage as the key to interrupting transmission. The reported numbers of vaccinations by NSEP sounded very impressive—over 324 million in the first two years (just 27 million vaccinations shy of the goal of 80 per cent vaccination coverage)—but outbreaks continued virtually unabated.

After a large epidemic of smallpox in Delhi that continued from December 1962 to the early months of 1963, the National Institute of Communicable Diseases (NICD) launched an independent assessment of NSEP. They found that coverage of vaccinations was closer to 60 per cent, rather than 80 per cent as reported by NSEP. In many places they found half the population was without primary vaccination. [11] Additionally, the success or "take rate" of primary vaccinations was only 86 per cent—in other words, one in seven of the people receiving vaccinations was not protected. Sometimes this

[10] Ibid., 8.

[11] H. M. Gelfand, "A Critical Examination of the Indian Smallpox Eradication Program", *American Journal of Public Health* 56, 1966, 1634–51.

was due to poor technique, other times it was due to bad vaccine. Liquid vaccine only retained its potency for forty-eight hours and needed refrigeration, which was often unavailable or inconsistent. The problem with keeping vaccine potent was important on two fronts: not only did impotent vaccine fail to stop smallpox, but it also contributed to widespread despair that smallpox would not be eradicated, leading leaders and villagers alike to shun vaccinators and the vaccination programme.

India's Third Five Year Plan ended in 1966, and the fourth did not begin until 1969 and during this time vaccination rates dropped substantially. However, in 1966 the World Health Assembly finally voted to create a global smallpox eradication programme, and nations all over the world committed themselves to set up eradication programmes as a priority. But for many political, domestic, and financial reasons, it was not until four years later, in 1970, that India up a WHO-assisted campaign.

Motivated by another large epidemic of smallpox in 1967 that was politically embarrassing, and the recognition of the unevenness in the quality of NSEP among the states, the central government made an important decision to essentially "nationalize" the smallpox programme. This was done by reclassifying the programme from being a "state issue" to a centrally sponsored "national programme". This meant the central government could impose standards of excellence and dictate programme strategy. When the Fourth Five Year Plan began in 1969, the central government could prod lethargic states into action and importantly, it could both evaluate weaknesses and mandate best practices. [12]

By the late 1960s, the mass vaccination programme was successful in achieving the highest vaccination coverage rates of any of the smallpox endemic countries in the world, but still it was unsuccessful at interrupting transmission. The concept of "density of susceptibles" later championed by Isao Arita of WHO had perhaps not been widely articulated, but it explained this apparent paradox. In a country of nearly 600 million, even a 90 per cent vaccine rate

[12] Brilliant, *Management of Smallpox Eradication in India*, 16.

still left 60 million susceptibles, more than enough to allow smallpox to spread dramatically.

The Indian teams learned many lessons during the NSEP's first decade, but because of problems ranging from poor vaccine quality to inadequate or substandard disease reporting, morale waned. The arrival of freeze-dried vaccine and the bifurcated needle, a simple device that made it possible for every villager to be a vaccinator, rejuvenating morale. The bifurcated needle looks like a flattened sewing needle with two prongs or tines that held exactly the right dose of vaccine. Freeze-dried vaccine administered with the bifurcated needle improved vaccination take rates to virtually 100 per cent. [13] Now that the team had both an effective vaccine and an easy way to administer it, what was needed was a bold new strategy and strengthened logistical and management tactics to attack the virus. As WHO became an active presence in the Indian eradication effort, with its first four field staff arriving in 1971, there would be many important moments that shaped and defined the effort leading up to the certification of eradication in India in 1977. [14] Three defining moments followed, changing the paradigm, awakening a campaign-like enthusiasm and surviving near catastrophe to emerge victorious.

Defining Moment: Changing the Mass Vaccination Paradigm into a Surveillance and Containment Strategy

Mass vaccination had worked in parts of Africa where population density was low. Compared with Africa, Asia boasted much higher population density so that even with a higher vaccination coverage, there remained a large number of people who had not been vaccinated, or who were also called *susceptibles*. [15] Isao Arita, another key player with the programme at WHO in Geneva, suggested that

[13] Brilliant, *Management of Smallpox Eradication in India*, 20.

[14] Ibid., 16.

[15] Ibid., 78–79.

the major problem in eradicating smallpox might not be the number of people vaccinated, but the *density of unvaccinated susceptibles*.[16]

In the early 1970s, there were half a million villages, a hundred and twenty million households, about 20 million new births each year, and at least ten million people travelling from one place to another at any given moment in India.[17] Even if a vaccinator thought she had achieved 100 per cent vaccination coverage, the 20 million unvaccinated newborns might have been enough to allow the disease to propagate. Add to that a more realistic rate of unvaccinated, and this is the key to understanding smallpox transmission. It is not the number of people vaccinated or the ratio of the people who have been vaccinated over the total population that is enough to explain transmission; it is the density of unvaccinated susceptibles—the number and clustering of susceptible people in a population.

A bold new strategy to replace the failing idea of mass vaccination was discovered by Bill Foege in Nigeria in 1966. In the midst of an epidemic and with insufficient vaccine, Foege, a visionary epidemiologist and physician, discovered an unexpected solution to the challenge of how to eradicate smallpox without vaccinating everyone.

Foege and his team were faced with a major smallpox outbreak during civil war in Nigeria, where they were living and working at that time. They could not get sufficient supplies of vaccine so Foege decided to prioritise, vaccinating only those people at highest risk, who had been directly exposed or were living a short distance away from active, infective cases. In this way, Foege and his team created a ring of vaccinated people around the virus and were able to stop the epidemic.[18]

Foege's discovery suggested that smallpox could be eradicated with a fraction of the number of vaccinations of mass vaccination—if those vaccinations were given in a targeted manner, to protect people most at risk, closest to each infectious case of the disease.

[16] Ibid.

[17] Basu, Jezek and Ward, *Eradication of Smallpox from India*, 2–6.

[18] W. Foege, Can Smallpox Be as Simple as 1-2-3?" *Washington Post*, 29 December 2002. Also see http://www.ph.ucla.edu/EPI/bioter/smallpoxsimple123.html.

This strategy was called "surveillance and containment" or selective epidemiologic control.[19] It meant focusing on interrupting the chain of transmission, rather than trying to vaccinate the entire population.[20] Later this technique was sometimes referred to as "ring vaccination".[21] This game-changing discovery in Africa was critical to the success of smallpox eradication in India.[22]

In 1973, Foege arrived in India on loan from the Centers for Disease Control (CDC) to help lead the WHO smallpox eradication programme there. The ring vaccination method worked very well in Indian trials and began to make its way into strategic planning in India as early as the 1970 Plan of Operations which paved the way for continued cooperation between NSEP and WHO. Though the strategy was sound, it relied on active case detection. But there was no active case detection in India yet; no one really knew how much smallpox was present in India or where it was. Under NSEP, India reported vaccinations, but there was no incentive to report cases of smallpox. In fact, at that time reporting a case of smallpox could have led to reprimand because an active case implied that mass vaccination had not worked. It is very likely that less than one case in ten was reported to central health authorities in India in 1967.[23] Slowly, the mass vaccination paradigm gave way to ring vaccination and a new strategy of surveillance and containment.

The goal of surveillance was to find every case of smallpox in the world. Containment meant isolating patients by creating a ring of immunity around them. It took three years to get from the idea of "surveillance" on paper, to effective surveillance in the field. Case reporting was improving in India, but as late as 1972 D. A. Henderson, reported, "case detection was inadequate, and the

[19] W. H. Foege, J. D. Millar and J. M. Lane, "Selective Epidemiologic Control in Smallpox Eradication", *American Journal of Epidemiology* 94, 1971, 311–15.

[20] Foege, Millar and Lane, "Selective Epidemiologic Control in Smallpox Eradication".

[21] Foege, "Can Smallpox be as Simple as 1-2-3?".

[22] Brilliant, *Management of Smallpox Eradication in India*, 16.

[23] R. N. Basu, "Smallpox Surveillance Status in India", *Journal of Communicable Diseases* 6, 1974, 974.

reporting systems were archaic; the importance of surveillance and containment was not appreciated."[24]

Later, an assessment component was added to the strategy of surveillance and containment. Health workers would go back to a random sample of villages or urban areas, usually one in every ten villages, and do systematic checks to see how accurate the disease surveillance and reporting were. Even after smallpox had been knocked out in an area, it was important for surveillance to continue in the absence of smallpox; eventually surveillance of chickenpox became a proxy measure to ensure that areas were still being searched monthly by smallpox workers. If the health workers were not finding cases of chickenpox, then it was likely they were not adequately searching for smallpox.

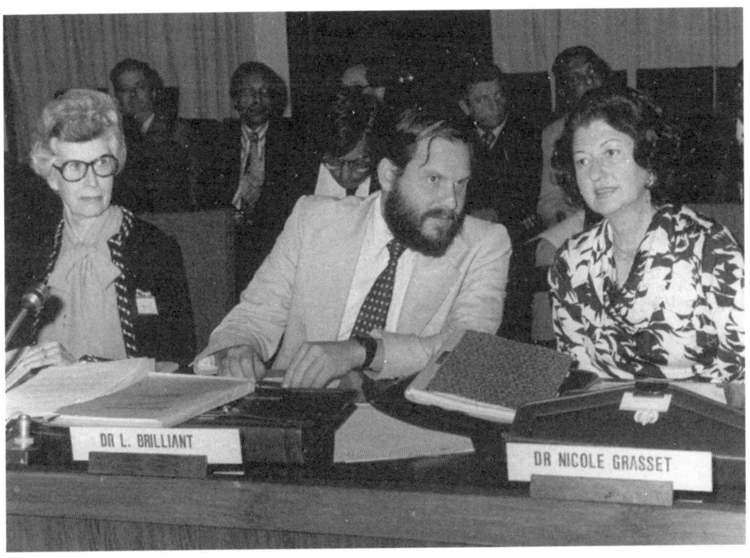

Figure 3.2: Dr Nicole Grasset and Dr Larry Brilliant from the WHO Central Team at the all India smallpox eradication review meeting, 1974.

Source: Photography provided by the author.

[24] D. A. Henderson, *Report on a Visit to the Smallpox Eradication Programme, India* (New Delhi: World Health Organization, SEA/SPX [restricted], June 1972).

Financial constraints remained a constant challenge throughout the eradication campaign. Though WHO and the Government of India provided increased financial and infrastructural contributions to the intensified campaign, the funding simply fell short of what was needed. The WHO smallpox staff were well aware of this and took their work very personally. Nicole Grasset, the charismatic smallpox eradication team leader in New Delhi and D. A. Henderson, head of the global programme in Geneva, spearheaded some of the first attempts to create "extra budgetary funds". In what was then unusual for WHO, they made direct appeals to a variety of civil society, corporate, multilateral and bilateral funding sources. They solicited a diverse group of funders including the Shah of Iran, UNICEF, the Swedish International Development Agency, OXFAM, Rotary and Lions clubs, the Tata Industries in India, as well as the People's Republic of China.[25] Indeed, WHO smallpox staff fund-raised over 90 per cent of smallpox funds in 1974–75.[26]

Incremental changes in approach were driven by faith that India could eliminate smallpox because Africa had done it. Additionally, the personal dedication of team members and committed leaders were fundamental to the ultimate success of the campaign. Nicole Grasset was one of the many who sacrificed so much to the mission of eradicating the first disease in history. D. A Henderson had seen a fearless Grasset head up relief missions flying vaccines for delivery in the midst of the Nigerian civil war. He knew he wanted Grasset running the WHO smallpox programme in the SEARO region that included Bangladesh, India, Nepal, Burma, Thailand and Indonesia among others.

When Grasset arrived in India, Indira Gandhi was Prime Minister. Mrs Gandhi had outlined a 20-point development programme for India and smallpox eradication was not on the list of her priorities. This translated into difficulties for Grasset, as smallpox team leader, to bring more staff, resources, and urgency to the programme in

[25] Sanjoy Bhattacharya, *Expunging Variola: The Control and Eradication of Smallpox in India* (Hyderabad: Orient Longman, 2006), 176.

[26] Brilliant, *Management of Smallpox Eradication in India*, 98.

India. Unafraid to break with WHO tradition, Grasset made a personal and direct appeal to India's Prime Minister, Indira Gandhi, appealing to her as both a leader of a country as well as a mother herself. She asked the Prime Minister to reconsider the global importance of smallpox. Grasset brought the Director-General of WHO, Halfdan Mahler, to India to meet with Prime Minister Gandhi to lobby to add smallpox as the 21st priority. Following this personal appeal, Gandhi accepted the logic that eradicating smallpox now would free up essential health services once they could be released from the smallpox campaign. Mrs Gandhi then wrote messages that motivated health workers throughout the country and continued to exchange letters with Grasset.[27] On 4 October 1974 Prime Minister Indira Gandhi released the following statement in support of the intensive search effort underway:

> Smallpox has been completely wiped out in most countries. India is unfortunately one of the small number where cases of smallpox still occur. Modern medicine can enable us to eradicate this disease. I'm glad to learn that an intensive three-month anti-smallpox campaign has been launched, particularly in the states of Uttar Pradesh, Madhya Pradesh, Bihar and West Bengal. This movement requires the fullest cooperation of all citizens. Parents especially must ensure that their children and indeed all young children in the neighbourhood are vaccinated against smallpox.[28]

This letter was written a year after the rest of the world, except for the sub-continent, had already eliminated *Variola major*. India was awakening to the magnitude of the problem and a programme built on this new strategy of surveillance, containment and assessment was about to be implemented.

Defining Moment: Awakening to the Magnitude of the Problem and the 1973 Autumn Campaign

After much negotiation, WHO and NSEP worked out a dual strategy. A nation-wide programme would begin, coordinated by

[27] Ibid., 97.

[28] For more details, see Bhattacharya, *Expunging Variola*, 202.

a "Central Assessment Team" comprised of WHO international epidemiologists and Government of India public health experts and under the leadership of M. I. D Sharma, Government of India's Commissioner of Health, and Nicole Grasset. India was divided into two major programme areas, one group of states were termed "endemic" and the other "low incidence" or, later, "non epidemic". Zdeno Jezek, a leading Czech epidemiologist fresh from the eradication of smallpox in Mongolia, was paired with C. K. Rao to maintain a continuing defence in the "non epidemic" states, while the rest of the Central Team paired off to focus on the four principal endemic states (Uttar Pradesh, Bihar, West Bengal and Madhya Pradesh). These four states accounted for nearly 80 per cent of India's smallpox in 1972.[29] The approach for Uttar Pradesh, Bihar, West Bengal and Madhya Pradesh included three phases. The first phase was an active case search in municipal areas during the summer of 1973 followed by a second phase of three weeklong, statewide searches that fall. WHO considered the searches from September through December most important. These door-to-door searchers of millions of homes required tens of thousands of vaccinators as well as the deputation of nearly all other health and family-planning workers—it was all hands on deck. The third phase was to be a mopping-up effort from January to December 1974 with the hope for a new year free of smallpox in 1975.[30] The findings from the autumn campaign were to provide the planning basis for the "final attack" phase in 1974. Ultimately, 150,000 workers made over one billion house calls and searched every house in India more than twenty times each, with an additional 10 per cent of homes visited a second time to assess the efficacy of case detection.

Officials in one state, Uttar Pradesh, initially refused to undertake a single-purposed search for smallpox only. They preferred an integrated approach such that the smallpox worker would perform other health activities, as well (i.e., malaria testing, condom and vitamin distribution). Adding all of these activities would have required more management than was available at that time and

[29] Brilliant, *Management of Smallpox Eradication in India*, 36.

[30] Ibid., 37.

diluted active case detection. Thanks to a well-known religious leader in the state who was very supportive of smallpox eradication, the smallpox team was able to meet with the Governor of Uttar Pradesh, A. A. Khan. The Governor realised that eradicating smallpox would free up significant resources to be available for malaria and family planning forever if eradication succeeded. His leadership in approving the short-term, single-purpose smallpox search campaign in Uttar Pradesh was very important to the quick success of the effort.

The search teams began intensified campaigns to overcome resistance to both disease reporting and vaccination. Search workers advertised everywhere: on elephants, on the backs of rickshaws and in movie theatres. Teams were equipped with "recognition cards"—printed photographs with the image of a smallpox-infected child. The goal was for everyone to know that smallpox was a terrible, disfiguring, deadly disease, that it could be conquered by vaccination, that there was a reward for reporting it and that it was going to be eradicated.

The reward was an important incentive that drastically improved reporting of cases. Search workers used a saffron coloured chalk-like local substance called "wet geru" to write on virtually every house in every village that a reward would be paid to anyone who found a case of smallpox. The programme first began with a reward of Rs 5 and moved it up to Rs 10, 25, 50 and eventually up to Rs 1,000 for every case reported. Every month, government search workers would enter a home, show the recognition card and ask if there was anyone who had a disease like that in the home. Occupants were told there was a reward for reporting a case of smallpox. The level of financial incentive became a metric for assessing the last time a home had been searched. If people reported having seen a search worker but stated that the reward was ten rupees when it had already grown to Rs 100, then it was assumed no vaccinator had visited since the time the reward was increased. This quantitative assessment let managers pinpoint programme deficiencies and take corrective action.

The first search was in West Bengal. Only 47 cases of smallpox were detected, but many districts were not searched due to flooding.[31] Programme management did not know whether a good search had found the few existing cases or a poor search had missed many. In October the massive follow-up search found only 143 infected villages, and Calcutta seemed to have far fewer infections than even the most optimistic had hoped.[32] West Bengal looked encouraging with less infections than anyone expected. Initial excitement gave way to shock as the searches continued in Uttar Pradesh and Bihar—the Indo-Gangetic plain and the historic heartland of smallpox—revealing more smallpox than anyone had thought existed in all of India.

In Uttar Pradesh the week before the search began the state reported 354 cases of smallpox occurring in twenty-one of the fifty-five districts of the state. On 15 October 1973, 27,000 workers set out to search 140,102 villages in one week.[33] By midday, telegrams were pouring in to programme managers at both the WHO smallpox unit and the Government of India. In Uttar Pradesh alone, smallpox cases were up seventeen times the amount reported the week before, almost 6,000 cases in forty-five districts. Bihar reported 614 new outbreaks with almost 4,000 cases. The search also began in Madhya Pradesh and workers reported 120 new outbreaks with 1,200 cases.[34] The week was number forty-two according to the WHO calendar, and the immediate spike in case reporting was obvious. The autumn campaign revealed a hidden epidemic; a shocking number of cases of smallpox had gone unreported, despite two solid years of work to improve reporting. This was a rude wakening to the size of the problem.

There were many reasons for the under-reporting of smallpox. Part of the problem was resistance to vaccination. Not everyone was eager or willing to be vaccinated, even with financial incentives. In addition to doubt about the efficacy of the vaccine, there were cultural and religious barriers to vaccination. In India, the goddess *Shitala Ma* for centuries was worshiped as the both the cause and

[31] Brilliant, *Management of Smallpox Eradication in India*, 42.

[32] Ibid.

[33] Ibid.

[34] Ibid., 43–44.

the cure of smallpox. In paintings and on sculptures she is depicted sitting on a donkey, carrying a winnowing bowl—a symbol of the Spring harvest—in her hands. Spring was the season when smallpox was at its worst. Shitala Ma was called various names like *Ma*, *Bashanto*, and *Mata* in different parts of India, but the general belief was the same: smallpox was the manifestation of her wrath, likely brought about by neglecting rituals in her honour.[35] Thus, the most common traditional prevention for smallpox was regular fulfillment of spiritual obligations to her. At the same time, however, Shitala Ma was regarded as having the power to mitigate smallpox and ease the pain. Her name means "the cool one" or "cooling mother".[36]

The temples of Shitala Ma thus became strategic observation posts for finding smallpox cases and offering vaccines. "Worship the Goddess, but also get the vaccine," became a slogan of choice for many a vaccinator. Among Indians living in rural areas, resistance to vaccine was a particular issue because vaccine was produced through scarification of the bellies of cows with Vaccinia or cowpox. After the virus grows on these cows, they were slaughtered to harvest quantities of vaccine. But since producing the vaccine caused the death of this animal so sacred to Hindus, it was hard to convince villagers to get vaccinated. Over time, Indian gurus and pundits began to support smallpox eradication, despite their mixed feelings about the way the vaccine was produced. India is a very religious country, with many strong religious communities of differing beliefs and customs. In fact, smallpox workers spent hundreds of hours talking to many priests, gurus, Jain monks, Buddhist monks, and others in an effort to reach an understanding that in the long run the eradication of smallpox would mean less vaccine and less killing of cows, and less human suffering. Ultimately, virtually every religious community in India approached by the smallpox programme gave their support.

[35] Ibid., 3.

[36] C. Maury, *Folk Origins in Indian Art* (New York: Columbia University Press, 1969).

Defining Moment: Surviving Near-Catastrophe with an Early Public-Private Partnership

By going house to house, smallpox workers provided accurate figures on India's smallpox burden and the autumn search campaign gave way to the planned phase three—what was to be the mopping up effort—in 1974. India and the world were awakening to the reality of smallpox in India. WHO strained to provide for the increased need for resources to allow the intensified campaign to continue. Then a critical bit of good luck brought additional funds. When The People's Republic of China declined to accept the $900,000 budgeted for assistance from the WHO in 1974, the Director-General requested and got agreement to transfer those funds to the India smallpox programme.[37] This allowed search operations to continue to improve, but that improvement in search quality led to finding more cases, and the officially reported incidence of smallpox then soared. Smallpox workers thought of this as an epidemic of reports, not as an epidemic of smallpox, but explaining to the press, the public and the politicians why, if things were going so smoothly, smallpox appeared to be reaching all time highs was very difficult. People did not care that the reporting had improved; it simply appeared that more people were getting smallpox inspite of—or because of—the change in strategy. And then things got even worse.

By March 1974, most of South India was free of smallpox, and one of the four endemic states—Madhya Pradesh—had been free of cases for months. Suddenly, community health workers began reporting cases of smallpox in parts of Madhya Pradesh that had been previously reported as smallpox-free.[38] Further investigation showed these were not simply previously undetected outbreaks; rather they were new importations of the disease from the state of Bihar. Other neighbouring states also reported fresh outbreaks. Investigators traced the source to Tatanagar, an industrial city in southern Bihar where many people went to find seasonal labour. Tatanagar was one of the few places where unskilled workers from

[37] Brilliant, *Management of Smallpox Eradication in India*, 44.

[38] Ibid., 46.

villages throughout India could come and get jobs; it was a magnet drawing workers from all over, and smallpox awaited them there. Struck with fever, many workers travelled the 200–500 miles home to Madhya Pradesh by train, where they then developed the rash of smallpox.[39]

The British had left a legacy of ubiquitous Indian railroads, which sadly became a contributing factor in spreading smallpox from Tatanagar. In fact, the Tatanagar railway station would soon become known as "the world's greatest exporter of smallpox" as "exports" from Tatanagar threatened to reinfect much of India that had already been freed of smallpox. Sick workers carried smallpox to five countries and 2,000 villages. This was a frightening epidemiological challenge. Thoughts of early victory over smallpox were crushed. Programme managers feared catastrophe.

Tatanagar was the headquarters of Tata Industry's TISCO subsidiary, an industrial steel and iron company. The area has been referred to as the Pittsburgh of India and had won several national awards as one of the most progressive cities in the country. While Tatanagar exported smallpox to much of India, the official weekly health records of the city showed only seven cases. The explanation soon became evident: health workers were hiding cases, suppressing reports of smallpox.

Soon newspapers focused international attention on the city and its corporate benefactor, Tata Industries, who had been unaware that the city they were so proud of had become home to a major international epidemic. Tata management was even more concerned to learn that a company doctor had failed to detect or report the largest hidden smallpox epidemic in the world. Tata, the Government of India and WHO entered into an agreement to extinguish the epidemic in Tatanagar. It was an early public-private partnership before such designations were widely used; WHO provided technical assistance, the government provided political leadership and Tata gave manpower, management and material. Tata's inputs, especially the dozens of high level skilled managers deputed to the programme, were essential to what became one of

[39] Ibid.

the most ambitious campaigns in the Indian smallpox programme. Within 72 hours, 50 doctors, 200 paramedical supervisors, 600 search workers, 50 vehicles and other services were mobilised to start the campaign.[40]

District magistrates and superintendents of police worked to quarantine the city. No one could leave or get on a train unless they were vaccinated. If they tried but refused vaccination, under the 1887 Bengal Immunity Act, they could be forcibly vaccinated. Containment, we had learned, worked well in Indian villages. But quarantining an entire modern Indian city was another level of difficulty. Fortunately, with the additional resources from Tata, containment held.

Tata went from unwitting host of an epidemic to a company deeply involved and committed to smallpox eradication. J. R. D. Tata, the head of Tata Industries suspended many routine business operations and sent dozens of managers and hundreds of assembly line workers to work with WHO and the Government of India and the state government of Bihar. It took six months of nonstop effort but what was once a name associated with despair among smallpox workers was transformed into an inspiring story of successful collaboration and cooperation. With Tatanagar no longer exporting disease to the rest of India, thoughts turned again to eradication and victory.

The "Virus" of Hope: Zero pox!

Smallpox epidemiologists would joke that there were two pox "viruses" circulating in India and South Asia in the mid 1970s—*Variola major*, which killed one in three who contracted it, and the equally contagious *Zeropox "virus"*, an infectious optimism that smallpox would be soon eradicated. This conviction that eradication was achievable, energised the smallpox teams. Word had gone out to governments and universities, institutes of health, and NGOs world wide—"come to India, come to Bangladesh and be part of history". Epidemiologists, infectious disease specialists, paediatricians,

[40] Ibid., 47.

history of medicine buffs, and would-be eradicators were drawn to witness or participate in an historic quest. In the midst of the Cold War, doctors from three dozen countries worked above and beyond their national interests and over international borders, bringing the best and brightest from UN agencies, government health ministries, international organisations, private companies, religious institutions and academe to support their Indian colleagues in the battle. People from all corners of the globe, from virtually every religion, continent, and all the colours of the rainbow put down their differences to work together to accomplish something much larger than any one of us individually. Smallpox eradication became a historic victory that says as much about the human capacity to overcome adversity as it does about the ability of epidemiology to conquer a single virus.

And it was the human element, the perseverance, the optimism, and the courage of the team that was continually tested. Moreover, there was to be one last reversal, one final test of resolve.

The last case of smallpox, *Variola minor*, occurred in Somalia. The last case of *Variola major* was Rahima Banu, who developed the disease on Bhola Island, in Bangladesh. But some of the most epic battles, the huge armies, the final skirmishes in the war against smallpox unfolded on the battlefield of the Gangetic plains of India. What was thought to be India's last known indigenous case of smallpox occurred on 17 May 1975. Manjho, an 8-year-old boy from Pachera village, Katihar District, Bihar developed rash on that day. As the government planned to celebrate both India's Independence Day and "independence from smallpox" on 15 August, WHO officials in Geneva and New Delhi took nothing for granted.

Neighbouring Bangladesh was still reporting smallpox and was in the throes of a civil war. Political instability in Bangladesh meant that surveillance and containment activities there were disrupted and that displaced people would likely flee toward bordering countries, like India. And then, almost as feared, a military coup in Bangladesh and the assassination of Prime Minister Mujibur Rahman created chaos, with massive migration into India. What was to have been a celebration of smallpox eradication in India instead became a rapid and determined mobilisation. A fresh series of searches was targeted at the India–Bangladesh border region. Nicole Grasset and D. A. Henderson were able to convince the Swedish International Development Agency to commit additional financial support to keep the programme going, especially the intensive surveillance along the borders through 1977.[41]

With such massive population movement from an endemic country, there had to be importations but fortunately the surveillance system worked. On 24 May 1975, the last known case of smallpox in India developed rash with fever. Saiban Bibi, a 30-year-old homeless Bangladeshi had come in contact with a case of smallpox in Thauri, Sylhet District of Bangladesh. She developed rash while living on the Karimganj railway station in Cachar district in Assam where she had come to beg for food. Containment was intense and effective. She was the last person to suffer from the historic scourge of smallpox in India, the historic home of this dreaded disease.

WHO and the Government of India had agreed that active case detection would continue for two years after what was thought to be the last case of smallpox, Then an independent international committee would certify the eradication of smallpox in India. Health ministry officials decided that all available staff would conduct two complete nationwide active search operations in October and December. They would record all cases of "rash with fever"—smallpox, chickenpox, scabies, measles and any other diseases that might indicate hidden smallpox cases. Scabs from these cases would be sent for lab analysis to assure the world that there was no more smallpox in India.[42] During this two-year period, several hundred thousand cases of smallpox like illness were investigated; most were chickenpox. None were smallpox. Maintaining the momentum of the smallpox eradication programme and keeping the teams well organised in the field, in the absence of cases of active smallpox through the two-year period of surveillance proved difficult, but ultimately rewarding. No additional cases of smallpox were ever found in India.

[41] Ibid.

[42] Bhattacharya, *Expunging Variola*, 219.

On 23 April 1977, the International Commission certified that smallpox had indeed been eradicated from India and with that put an exclamation point at the end of one of the most stirring campaigns in the history of medicine and public health.

4

The Last Challenge: The Horn of Africa

Ciro de Quadros

Introduction

This chapter describes some of my experiences while I worked for the World Health Organization (WHO) in Ethiopia during the smallpox eradication programme. By coincidence, I recently arrived from Addis Abeba, where I presided over a Technical Advisory Group that reviewed the polio eradication initiative in the Horn of Africa. Therefore, some of my memories were refreshed during this last visit and it was quite interesting to observe the tremendous changes that took place in the country over the last twenty-five years. This chapter is illustrated by figures and pictures to describe some of the experiences we had during the course of the six years I was stationed there.

Ethiopia is a country with approximately 77 million people and 1.2 million sq km. It is the second largest country in Africa and in 1970 had a population of 25 million, mostly dispersed in the rural countryside. Infrastructure was rudimentary in all respects, including communications, schools and health facilities. At that time it had less than 5,000 km of all-weather roads, access was quite limited and difficult (Map 4.1). The country has a very challenging topography with the central highlands, the southwest forest area, the southeast Rift Valley and the Ogaden Desert. Addis Abeba, the capital of Ethiopia, is the third highest capital in the world. The country was divided into fourteen provinces and the provinces were divided into *awrajas* (districts) and the awrajas into *woredas* (sub-districts).

MAP 4.1: Topography and road system in Ethiopia, 1970

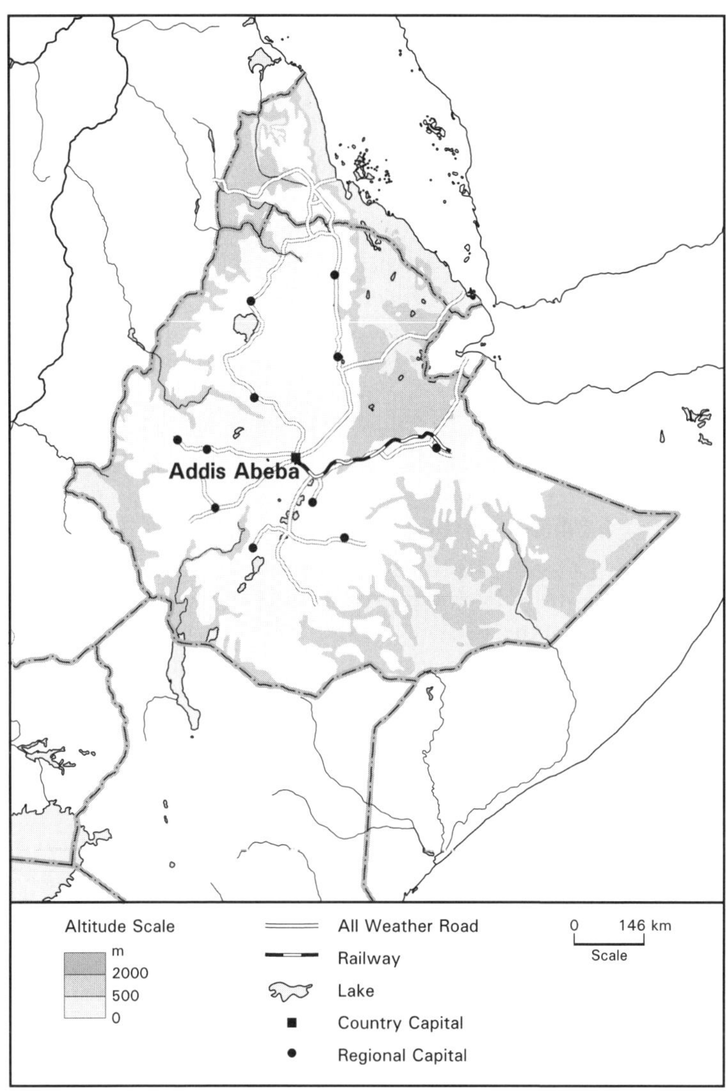

Source: © World Health Organization.

In 1970, Ethiopia was still a monarchy under the Emperor Haile Selassie, with feudal landlords and the Ethiopian Coptic Church dominating most of the countryside. Travelling in the interior of the country felt as if you had stepped into the Middle Ages; people lived in small hamlets and shared their huts in the evenings with their livestock.

At that time this country of 25 million people had only eighty-four hospitals, sixty-four health centres, less than 400 physicians and only about 2,800 other health staff. Each province had a health department, called the Provincial Medical Department which was staffed by a medical officer, usually a European physician; particularly in the south-western provinces the health departments were staffed by Swedish physicians. The other health departments were staffed with health officers that received training in a school of public health in the capital of Begemdir province in the north of the country. This school graduated what some call "Chinese barefoot doctor". These graduates were well prepared to deal with the major morbidity in their area of responsibility, including performing minor surgeries, obstetrics, paediatrics and general medical care. Besides the health officer, the Provincial Medical Department had a sanitarian and some assistant nurses. This gives you an idea of the poor health infrastructure existing in the country at that time.

The Launching of the Programme

In 1970, smallpox vaccination was essentially unknown by the population and variolation—the practice of inoculating material from an infected smallpox patient into a healthy individual—was used in various regions of the country.

Interestingly, the government had absolutely no interest in the eradication of smallpox, and like many other countries, argued that Ethiopia did not have a smallpox problem. There was an Anti-Epidemic Service in Addis Abeba which was directed by a Greek physician, named Dr Papaioannu, who affirmed to the Emperor that Ethiopia did not have smallpox. As a result, when Dr D. A. Henderson, from the WHO, and his team went to Addis Abeba to plan the eradication programme they estimated that very few cases would be found. They went through all the records and came to the conclusion that smallpox was very rare in Ethiopia. This led them to believe that eradication could be achieved with fewer resources than in fact later came to be necessary.

Most of the resources of the Ministry of Health at that time were devoted to malaria eradication. The malaria advisers were boycotting the smallpox eradication programme because they viewed smallpox as a competition to their programme. Because of the boycott, when Dr D. A. Henderson presented the smallpox initiative to ministry officials he was greeted very coldly. The situation only changed when he met an Austrian physician called Kurt Weithaler who was the Director of the Imperial Bodyguard Hospital. Dr Weithaler was very well connected with the Emperor. This connection helped the Minister of Health to move forward with the programme, under the orders of the Emperor.

Nevertheless, because officials were not very enthusiastic and because it was thought that smallpox was not a problem, they assigned a small number of personnel to the programme—around twenty-five. Dr D. A. Henderson succeeded in increasing the number of people working on the programme by reaching an agreement with the American Peace Corps. This added seventeen volunteers to the programme for a period of two years. This arrangement lasted for about four years, with yearly replacement of the volunteers. Subsequently, the Japanese International Cooperation Agency (JICA) provided a few volunteers, some worked as surveillance officers and others helped manage the radio communication system and the car repair shop. The Austrian government also provided four volunteers to operate as surveillance officers.

After training the staff assigned to the programme on the techniques of surveillance and containment, the programme was launched at the beginning of 1971 in the four provinces of the south and south-western part of the country which had a slightly better infrastructure.

Ethiopia was the first country in the world to start the programme from day one with the strategy of "surveillance and containment", not mass vaccination. Mass vaccination was never used. The operational plan that was put together consisted of the search for cases and outbreaks (surveillance), followed by the vaccination of all contacts of the cases in the various chains of transmission (containment). At the start of operations there were only six Land Rovers, four deployed to each of the four provinces, and the rest to two surveillance officers (one Ethiopian sanitarian and one American Peace Corps volunteer) to look for cases and start the vaccination of contacts.

Of course, the organisation of a surveillance system in a country without an adequate health infrastructure was a challenge. We requested that all the available health facilities (hospitals, health centres and stations) report suspected cases by making personal contact with all the directors of the provincial medical departments, local governors and officials in all districts and sub-districts.

We also used a novel strategy of case finding through schools and marketplaces. The surveillance officers would visit these places and show a picture of a smallpox patient, asking: “Has anybody seen a case of smallpox similar to this one?” To our surprise almost everybody would answer: “I saw a case!” This strategy was very successful as in the first two to three years of operations transmission was interrupted in the four provinces.

The Expansion of the Programme

By mid-1972 we received additional vehicles and camping equipment. We were then able to start organising the other provinces because until that time the two individuals had been working with the few resources they could find. If a car that would take them to investigate an outbreak was available they would go if not, they could not go. Sometimes they would go on foot. In the first three to four years of the programme we walked like I had never walked in my life! Still today when I am invited to walk my answer is: “I have walked all the miles I had the right to in Ethiopia, I have no miles left”! Indeed, it was very difficult to walk because it was usually in the mountainous areas and the hamlets were located far from one another.

When Dr D. A. Henderson talked to the Malaria Director and asked for logistical assistance he was informed that the malaria programme had no cars. This was very interesting because we knew that the malaria eradication had received over forty vehicles before we arrived. Later on the WHO Malaria Advisor said that when they heard that the smallpox programme was going to start, they drove all the cars to a town near the desert, a town called Nazareth, to hide them and avoid lending the cars. It is unbelievable but it happened!

Furthermore, the Greek Director of the Anti-Epidemic Service began a boycott by telling the Emperor and the Minister of Health that cases of smallpox were reported only after WHO started the programme. He argued that these were not smallpox cases and that the programme was not vaccinating enough people. He was proposing that the programme be stopped.

By the end of 1971, when the first year of the programme was completed, we had reported over 26,000 cases! Even Dr D. A. Henderson was suspicious and wrote to us asking if we were "reporting rumours", because this was totally unexpected.[1] However, we had an epidemiological record for every case reported. The system established registered the patient as well as their entire family. It also included the number of contacts that were vaccinated in the outbreak area. All this information was analysed and published in the *Weekly Surveillance Bulletin* that was a feedback to those involved in the programme as well as to all health officials in the country.

The photograph Figure 4.1 was taken during my first trip to the southern province of Illubabor, on the border with Sudan. We were with the district Governor and the Health officer in charge of the Health Centre in the area. Accompanying me is a Peace Corps volunteer who often carried a violin and used to play at the campsite at night. It was quite an experience to hear this very nice violin in the middle of the jungle!

The photograph Figure 4.2 illustrates the lack of roads. This is a path on the border of Ethiopia and Sudan in the area where the Blue Nile crosses the border coming from its source, Lake Tana. The Blue Nile goes into Sudan and meets with the White Nile in Khartoum, forming the river Nile.

[1] Letter from Dr D. A. Henderson.

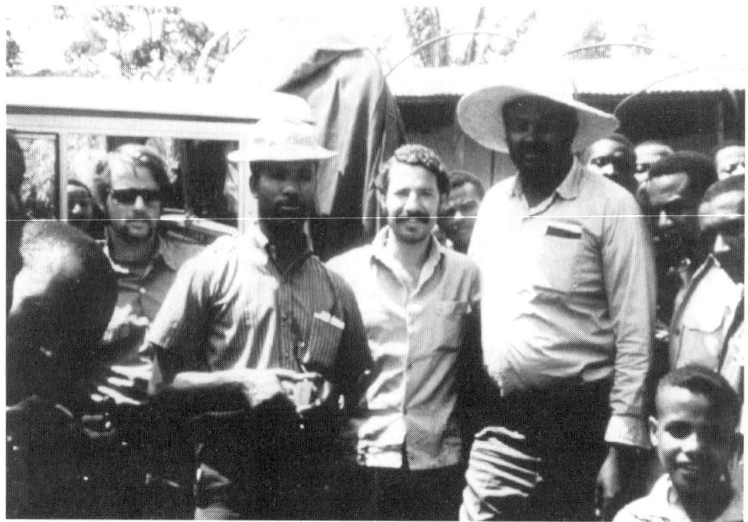

FIGURE 4.1: Southern province of Illubabor, on the border with Sudan.

Source: Photograph provided by Mark Strassburg.

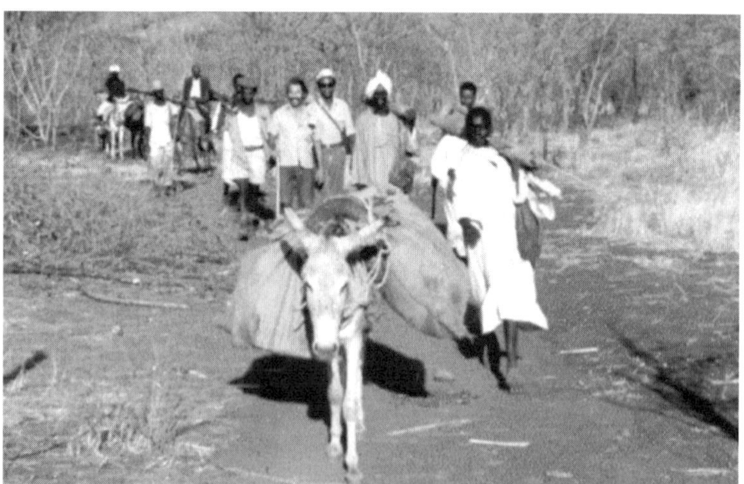

FIGURE 4.2: Ethiopia and Sudan border, 1972.

Source: © World Health Organization.

During one of our outbreak investigation trips we walked for twenty-six days going from village to village. We started the trip with the chief of the area and his three donkeys carrying our equipment. There were about five people in our group. The river bed was dry and to get water we had to dig and wait for it to come. To our dismay, the chief would say "the first water to come out is for the donkeys because if not they will die". We would ask, "Where is the next village?" and they would reply: "Over that hill"[2].

The interesting part of this trip was that we started with about five people and ended the trip with more than thirty. This was the first time that foreigners came to that area. In each village that we stopped people would join us and go to the next village. We had the opportunity to map this entire area and provided the Ethiopian Map Institute with copies since at that time they did not have a clue of the layout of that area.

At some point during the trip, we unknowingly crossed the Sudanese border and were arrested and held for one day at the police station. We started a hunger strike which I think frightened somehow the Chief of the police station because soon after the police released us. This release avoided a big fight. When we returned to Ethiopia, the Ethiopians were coming well-armed to rescue us.

The photograph Figure 4.3 illustrates some of the bridges that we crossed. In some rivers we had to pull the cars with winches so that the cars would essentially float during the crossing.

The Transition Challenges

In 1974 we had a transitional period when, a revolution led by the military, overthrew Emperor Haile Selassie.

It was of course a very difficult period in the country and all UN operations were stopped, with the exception of our programme, because if we had stopped at that time it would have been disastrous. We received permission to stay in the country but the Peace Corps volunteers were withdrawn and we were left without their help. However, since additional resources were forthcoming from the

[2] Personal communication.

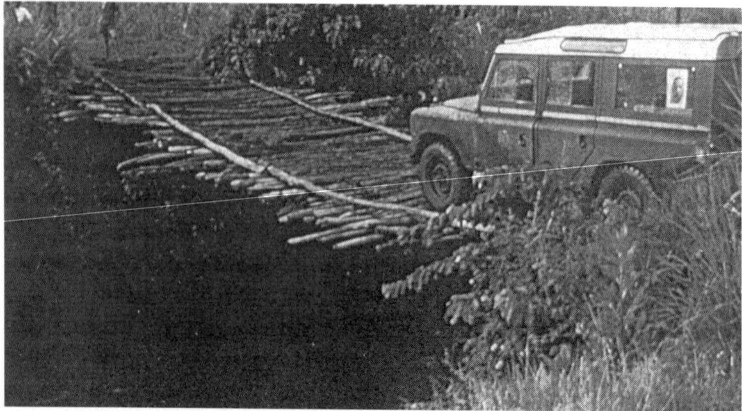

FIGURE 4.3: River crossing in Ethiopia.

Source: © World Health Organization.

WHO we were able to get more nationals. We also hired local people in addition to the ones that the government had assigned to the programme. Many senior health staff from Ethiopia were hired, including a very competent Ethiopian, to be the counterpart of the Director of the programme, and another to be my counterpart as the Chief Epidemiologist. In each province we started the hiring of more senior Ethiopians, with the programme being 'nationalised'. It was the best phase of the programme.

During this transition period there were many challenges. There was a time when the government decided that no private aircrafts could fly in the country because they wanted to avoid the escape of people from the country. There were also issues related to currency flowing out of the country. But again we came to an agreement with the government to keep our programme going. At this point we had already received additional resources, including aerial support with five helicopters and a couple of fixed wing aircrafts. We also had the support of C47 aircrafts that would carry jet fuel at any given time to the bases where the helicopters were located. These resources were made available in part because smallpox had been eradicated in India and Bangladesh, releasing both financial and human resources to areas where smallpox was still endemic.

The government allowed us to fly the helicopters and aircrafts on condition that we carry an army official with us. This was agreed to since the programme could benefit from their knowledge of the local language—they could serve as interpreters between the staff and local population. This arrangement satisfied all parties and we continued the programme with no major difficulties.

The shaded part of Map 4.2 shows the areas that still had smallpox transmission during this period. They were mostly in the highlands, an extremely difficult area to work in. The people inhabiting these areas are the most traditional Coptic Christians. These areas, controlled by the Ethiopian Coptic Church priests and the population, were very resistant to vaccination. Sometimes teams would stay for days in the villages and would sometimes vaccinate only the chief of the village and maybe one other person and leave with very few individuals vaccinated. All in spite of the fact that transmission was occurring.

Resistance came to the point where people would expel surveillance officers from the villages by any means necessary—sticks and stones and even a hand grenade was thrown as a helicopter was taking off from a hamlet.

We used to distribute health workers in the area by dropping them off in the morning and picking them up late in the afternoon. Whenever helicopters came to a village the people would be very excited because it was something they had never seen. The first time we flew a helicopter to one village the blade was broken by a big stick carried by a peasant. We were stuck in this village for a couple of days until we could get another helicopter to pick us up. Children would also throw stones when the helicopters were taking off. On one occasion when the pilot was taking off an individual threw what was thought to be a stone, but it was actually a hand grenade that exploded under the helicopter. Fortunately the pilot and passengers were able jump out of the helicopter before it was completely destroyed and nobody was injured. The hand grenade was old, from the times of the Italian invasion and could still be bought in the market places. The individual who threw the hand grenade was a priest who wanted to "defend the village against the heretics want to change our religion".

Map 4.2: Ethiopia: Awraja areas (shaded) in which cases of smallpox were reported, 1974–76

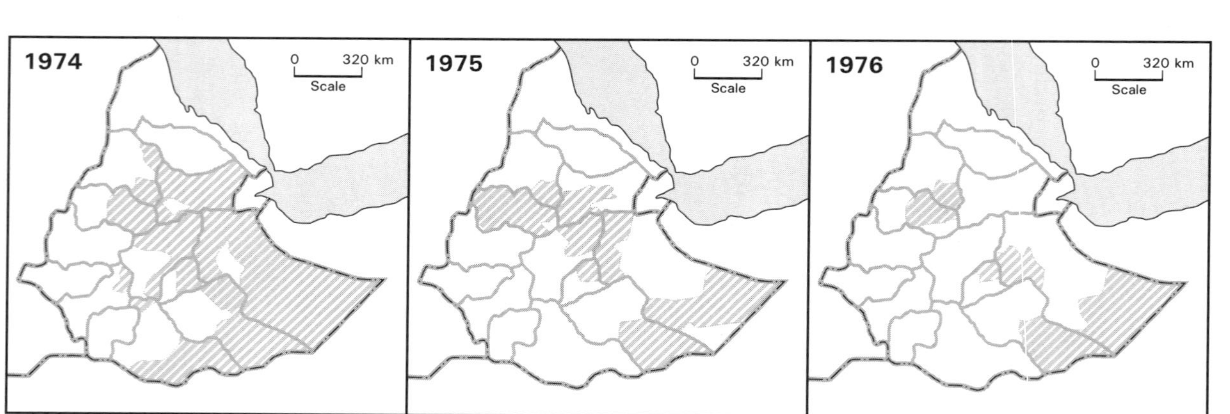

Source: © World Health Organization.

Another interesting vignette also happened in the highland area, just south of the Blue Nile gorge, one of the most beautiful areas of Ethiopia. As I mentioned before, we used to go to the marketplaces and schools and show pictures of smallpox patients, asking if anybody knew of similar cases in their village. We would give a reward of ten Ethiopian dollars if such a report turned out to be a smallpox case.

On one such occasion, when we visited a market place on the southern edge of the Blue Nile gorge we received a report from an individual who knew of a smallpox case. We immediately flew him by helicopter to his village where he introduced us to his young wife who had smallpox. We started the epidemiological investigation and the containment vaccination by keeping one vaccinator at the door of the house to either vaccinate those who entered, or to deny entrance to those who refused vaccination. Afterwards we returned to the market place and gave him the ten dollar reward in plain view. This event nearly created a war with the people from across the northern part of the gorge, where the wife came from. News spread that the reporter of the case had sold his wife to the foreigners. Her family was attempting to rescue her. You can imagine the commotion that went through that village until this was sorted out.

As the programme proceeded, cases started diminishing. The last cases in 1976 were in the highlands, which was populated by the Ahmara, a very difficult area to work, due to refusal of the people to vaccination. At the same time transmission continued in the Ogaden desert, the nomadic area bordering Somalia. This was the scene of several events that made the programme extremely difficult.

Today, thirty years later, the polio eradication initiative is struggling with similar problems in the same region. Nowadays the problem appears to be exacerbated. Thirty years ago there was an established government in Somalia with whom it was possible to have a dialogue. Today there is no government, only clans fighting each other and it has proven to be an extremely difficult place to operate.

At that time there were guerrillas in Eritrea, which was then a province of Ethiopia. However, the programme in Ethiopia worked with the guerrillas, which accepted and somehow facilitated the epidemiological work and the containment vaccination. With the help of the guerrillas transmission was interrupted in Eritrea without many difficulties. In the Ogaden, however, the Somali guerrillas harassed the surveillance teams and in several instances kidnapped these individuals and took them to Modagishu. Eventually, after negotiations, they would release the workers, but would keep the vehicles and communication equipment.

The Final Phases

The graph below (Figure 4.4) shows the number of cases of smallpox from 1971 to 1976. In 1971 there were 25,000 cases. By 1972 the number had been reduced to 16,000 and to about 5,400 in 1973. In 1974 and 1975 cases remained relatively stable at around 4,000, diminishing to 915 cases in 1976 with the last case in August of that year. The graph also shows the monitoring of the number of districts or sub-districts that were harbouring transmission at any given time. The monitoring of the programme during this last phase was through the number of affected districts or villages, which were then followed up during the ten weeks following the last detected case. If no further cases were detected during that period, the village or district was taken off the list of affected areas.

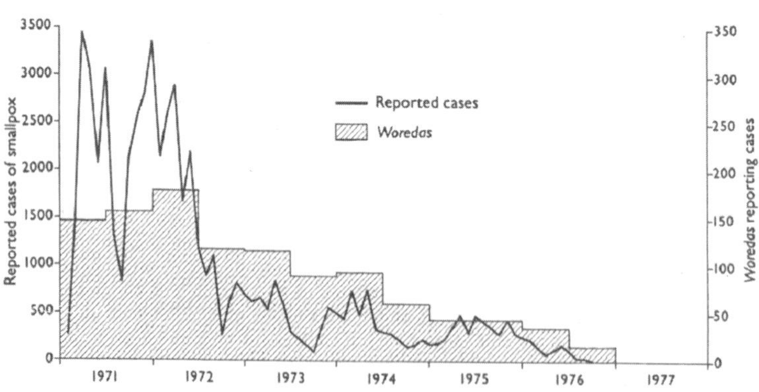

FIGURE 4.4: Number of reported cases of smallpox, by month and number of woredas, reporting cases, by six month periods, 1971–76

The photographs below show the operation in the Danakil Depression. The families lived in small huts (Figure 4.5) and the vaccinator had the vaccine protected from the sun with a hat (Figure 4.6). Fortunately the smallpox vaccine was heat stable and therefore worked well in the heat of the desert. This area also presented several obstacles as it was controlled by a Sultan who did not recognise the authority of the Central Government. This Sultan controlled all the areas known as the Danakil Depression, inhabited by the Afar and Issa tribes, bordering Djibouti. The first time we visited this area we were chased out. Only after discussions with the Sultan and receiving his agreement that the operation could be launched, were we able to work in the area. From this point onward the work went smoothly and was appreciated by the population in the area.

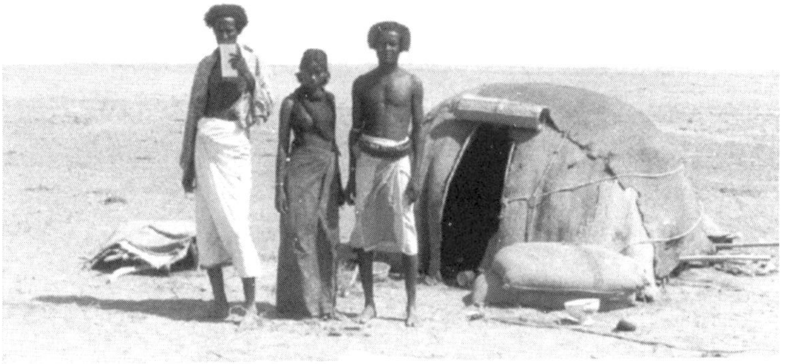

FIGURE 4.5: Danakil Depression: A family in front of their small hut.

Source: Photograph provided by the author.

Figure 4.7 shows the last case in Ethiopia in the village of Dimo in the south-western part of the Ogaden, where the child was living at the time. This area remains inhabited for only a few weeks in the year, as these pastoral, nomadic people roam the countryside, following the rain. They make fences out of torn bushes so that lions, hyenas and other wild animals cannot enter their houses (Figure 4.8). All these areas were mapped by the surveillance teams, which could then trace the location of the nomads at any given time.

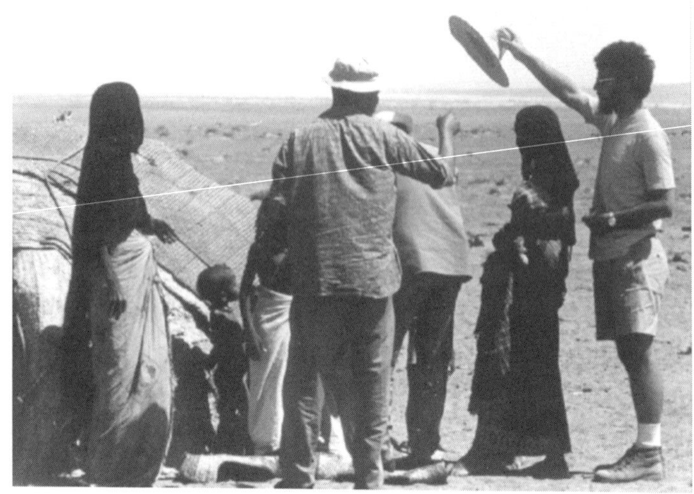

FIGURE 4.6: Work in the Danakil Depression.

Source: Photograph provided by the author.

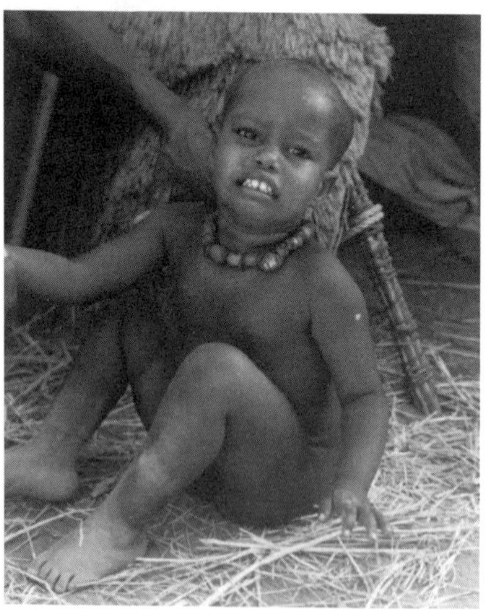

FIGURE 4.7: Last case of smallpox in Ethiopia.

Source: Photograph provided by the author.

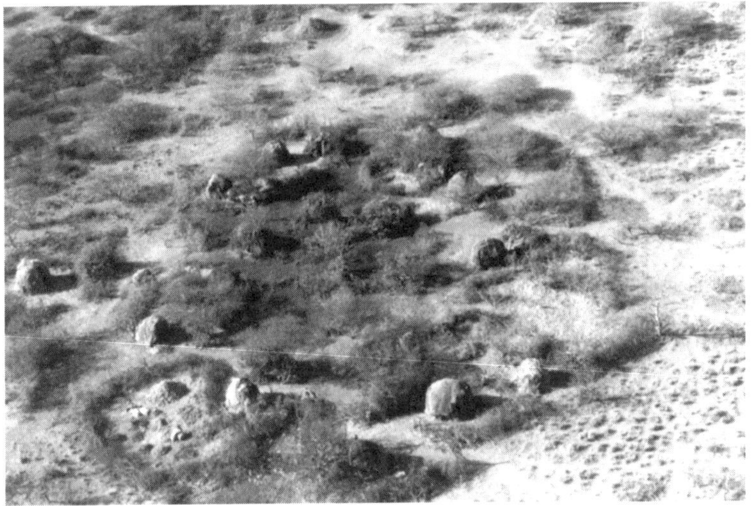

FIGURE 4.8: Village of Dimo in the south-western part of the Ogaden.

Source: Photograph provide by the author.

The surveillance officer/vaccinator was dropped off by the helicopters in a given hamlet and two or three days later was picked up several kilometres away in another hamlet. He would walk for two or three days, following the pattern of the nomads and looking for cases and/or tracing the chains of smallpox transmission and vaccinating contacts of cases. This is how we came to meet a little girl by the name of Amina Salat. She was a mild case, as she had been vaccinated during the incubation period.

We thought that she was the last case of smallpox in the world and were very excited, in spite of the fact that we strongly suspected transmission on the Somali side of the border. We insisted with Geneva that there were cases in Somalia, but Dr D. A. Henderson and his team in Geneva kept telling us that there were no cases in Somalia, as reported by the WHO representative and his team. Nevertheless, the people living in the Ogaden did not really know that a border existed. It was a virtual border, created somewhere in Europe after the Second World War, when somebody traced a line somewhere in the Horn of Africa, dividing the area inhabited by the same people into what is now known as Ethiopia and Somalia. Therefore, during any given year, these people would travel on both sides of the border taking their cattle and camels to wherever they could find grass and water.

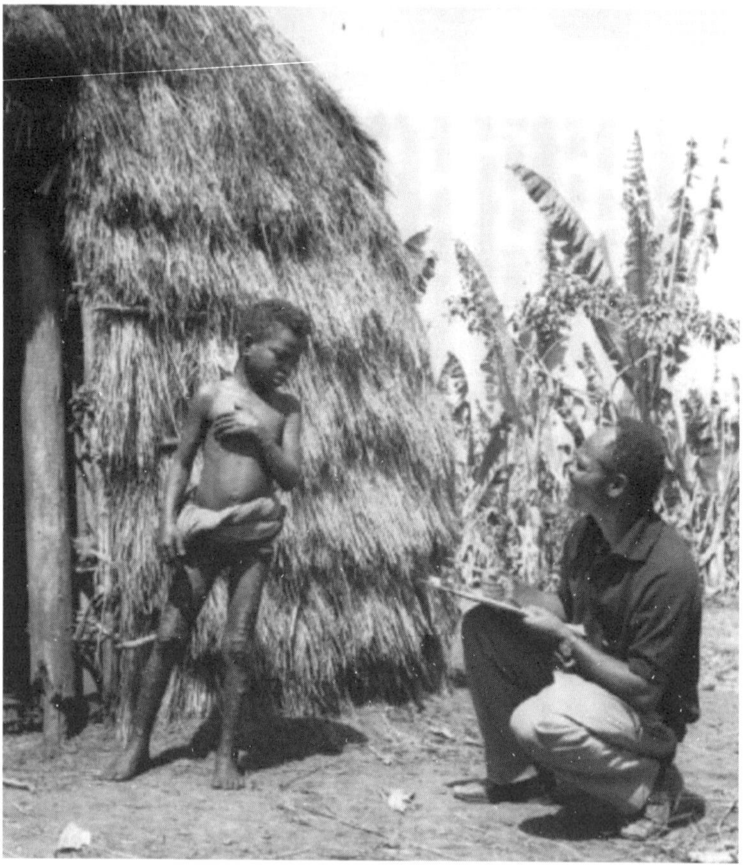

FIGURE 4.9: A surveillance officer investigates a case of smallpox in southern Ethiopia.

Source: © World Health Organization.

As the case in Dimo was thought to be the last case in the world, many people came to see the area and photograph the case. Dr D. A.

Henderson came, along with reporters from *National Geographic*, and we had a party at the end of the day. During the party we received a report of smallpox in a village north of the Ogaden, which brought a cloud over the celebration. The next morning we flew to the village from where the report originated and found out that the case was chickenpox.

The operations in the Ogaden were extremely difficult and dangerous. The gentleman who provided the fixed wing aircrafts was Count Von Rosen, from Sweden, a famous humanitarian. He was eventually killed when guerrillas attacked the Governor's compound in Gode, the capital of the province of Ogaden, less than a mile from the smallpox camp, which was not attacked! One helicopter pilot was also kidnapped and the WHO received a note that the guerrillas wanted 40,000 Ethiopian dollars for his release. Eventually the pilot was released without payment of the ransom, which was already on the way when the pilot was freed.

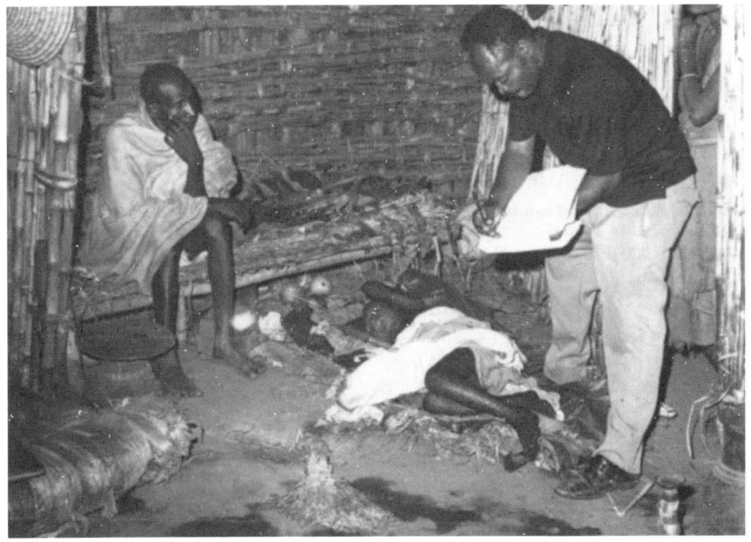

FIGURE 4.10: A severe case of smallpox is recorded by a surveillance officer.

Source: © World Health Organization.

The programme in Ethiopia lasted six years with a lot of excitement. When you are working under such circumstances, with such a goal to be achieved, you do not even realise the real situation you are in. I only realised the extent of the situation when I left Ethiopia and read in the international press the daily dispatches about the war in the Horn of Africa. And apparently, in spite of these incidents, the general population appreciated the work that was being done and in general collaborated with the programme.

The paramount factor that made the programme successful was the incredibly high quality and dedication of the people assigned to the programme. They were trained in basic epidemiological principles for the eradication of smallpox and disease control and were integrated with the rudimentary primary health care infrastructure existent in the country, which received support from the programme. In addition, during the period of the revolution, the government closed all the schools for a period of one year to launch an education campaign with the high school and university students. Approximately 60,000 students were sent to the countryside to indoctrinate the population on the aims of the revolution. At the start of this initiative they did not have adequate logistical support. Our programme collaborated with them by providing some logistical support and in return they looked for smallpox cases in their assigned areas. With this we added thousands of individuals to our surveillance network. They also collaborated in enlightening the population on the benefits of vaccination to stop transmission of the disease.

The Funding of the Programme

Funds received for this programme was about $14.3 million. The WHO mobilised $13 million and most of that was used by the helicopter operation because was very expensive. We had five helicopters flying, each one flying seven to eight hours a day which greatly increased the cost of this operation. The government provided the salaries of the people they assigned to the programme and in many instances collaborated on logistical support in the different provinces.

The Somalia Setback

Then, at the beginning of January 1977, the news came about an outbreak in Somalia came in. I did not work in Somalia; therefore I cannot talk much about that. I had left Ethiopia in the middle of January 1977, and one day after arriving in Geneva a cable arrived from Somalia reporting cases of smallpox. There was much turmoil in Geneva as Dr D. A. Henderson and his team immediately started looking for the answer. Unbelievably, in a few short weeks they were able to organise an airlift from Europe that brought much needed vehicles and camping equipment so that the teams could respond to the outbreak. Several experienced veterans of the operations in India, Bangladesh and Ethiopia were deployed immediately and between February and August the transmission was interrupted.

Eradication of Diseases after Smallpox

Smallpox was the first disease ever to be eradicated in the history of mankind. It provided us with important lessons that can be applied in public health in general and in disease control and eradication in particular. In 1981, four years after I had moved to Washington DC to work for the Pan American Health Organization (PAHO), which is the regional office of the WHO for the Americas, I suggested to Dr D. A. Henderson, who was then the Dean of the School of Hygiene and Public Health at Johns Hopkins University in Baltimore, the eradication of poliomyelitis from the Western hemisphere. His answer was: "No way!"[3] Nevertheless, we had observed that Cuba had eradicated polio in the early 1960s as soon as the oral polio vaccine developed by Albert Sabin became available. They accomplished this by implementing mass vaccination days, twice a year. In 1980 Brazil, which is a huge country, applied the same strategy and vaccinated approximately 20 million children under five in one day, which was unheard of at that time. Later on, this strategy was implemented in China, India and elsewhere where they still continue vaccinating millions to this day. The strategy utilised in Brazil almost stopped transmission of polio and showed that if

[3] Personal communication.

applied correctly elsewhere in the Americas, transmission could be interrupted in the entire continent.

Therefore, I went back to Dr D. A. Henderson mainly because I thought it would be very difficult to start another eradication programme without his support. This time I argued that the data from Brazil showed that the job could be done if resources were made available. This time his answer was: "I'm going to learn Spanish and help you".[4] We stopped polio transmission in the Americas in 1991 with Dr D. A. Henderson's help, although, he never did learn Spanish!

It is important to note that during the polio eradication in the Americas we applied several lessons learned from the smallpox programme. First, you need to have a very clear vision of where you want to go and what the real objective is that you want to achieve. Second, the strategy has to be very well articulated and stated in a simple way that is understood by everybody involved in the programme, from headquarters to the field level. Third, and most importantly, you need to have all the resources you need to do the job. Fourth, you need strong and good management and supervision at all levels, with adequate surveillance in place from the outset of the programme. Fifth, you need to analyse the data coming from the field to adapt the strategy to every situation that may arise. And last, but not least, you need to provide feedback to all parties involved.

These are lessons that many people do not utilise in their disease control/eradication programmes these days. It is noticeable that the polio eradication initiative has had a chronic funding gap since its inception and this is one of the various reasons why the initiative is faltering. There are not sufficient resources to do the job. If you look at the WHO documents it often describes a funding gap of approximately $500 million every year. Before we started the polio eradication programme in the Americas in 1985, we calculated how much it would cost, what could the governments of the endemic countries provide and what was needed in addition to support these governments. We found that we would have to mobilise about $120 million, for a programme estimated to last five years. The

[4] Personal communication.

announcement of the PAHO initiative, in May 1985, was only made when we had the assurance that funds would be made available, with firm commitments from the potential partners, which were Rotary International, UNICEF, USAID and the Inter-American Development Bank.

If future eradication initiatives are launched, and I believe that there are other diseases that could be eradicated, such as measles and rubella, for instance. I hope that the future leaders of those initiatives will follow some of the smallpox eradication lessons.

5

Innovation as an Integral Part of Smallpox Eradication: A Fieldworker's Perspective

Alan Schnur

Introduction

Smallpox eradication is acknowledged as one of the greatest public health achievements. Many books have been written, in many countries, on the management and technological basis of the programme. However, the increased level of effort to move from a control programme to an eradication programme is frequently under-estimated. For an eradication programme there is almost no margin for error. If you make a mistake, leave an area uncovered, the virus will find the weak link and attack there. A success rate of 95 per cent may be very good for control programmes, but it is not good enough for eradication. The increased efforts to move from a control programme to an eradication programme required an immense, high quality contribution from all programme participants—from senior leaders in the WHO headquarters, to regional and country leaders, to field-workers serving as mid-level managers at district level, or as vaccinators and surveillance staff at village level.

What was remarkable about the smallpox eradication effort was not that a few talented senior staff drove the programme through review and analysis of data, and mobilising expert advice at international meetings, although this did happen, but that average fieldworkers at all levels throughout the programme felt empowered, indeed felt responsible, to make technically sound and locally relevant innovations based on their field judgement and experiences, and inputs from national colleagues.

The full mobilisation, empowerment and involvement of fieldworkers as essential contributors to the smallpox effort created tremendous creative energy within the programme which resulted in many important, even critical, innovations and made an essential contribution to the eradication effort.

This chapter will review the culture of empowerment and innovation which percolated throughout and drove the smallpox eradication effort, from the perspective of a fieldworker working at province or district level and below. The first section will look at this aspect from the programmatic perspective, based on the review of literature. The second section will provide a personal perspective of the programme, based on experiences of the author during the smallpox eradication work in Ethiopia, Uttar Pradesh (U.P.) in India, Bangladesh and Somalia during the period 1971–78. Varied sources of information have been used for this chapter, including published articles and books, the author's recollection, original field notebooks and unpublished newsletters.

Selected innovations, which increased the efficiency and effectiveness of the smallpox effort, will be reviewed with emphasis on innovations originated by fieldworkers (both WHO and national staff) in the field. The chapter will illustrate that these innovations were not accidental events, but the result of a conscious policy and effort of programme management to convey to fieldworkers that their contributions and problem-solving efforts were essential elements of the successful eradication effort.

Field staff who felt, and were made to feel, that their contribution was essential to the success of the programme put in tremendous efforts to solve problems and find creative solutions to bottlenecks, with steps often taken to make the programme more efficient to save resources and time. Mid-level WHO epidemiologists in turn fully involved lower level and mid-level national staff in the programme, and included the national staff's ideas in discussions with senior government staff and in problem-solving.

Along with the atmosphere of empowerment of field staff went a strong culture of assessment and evaluation of efforts and dissemination of the results. Innovations were tried by fieldworkers but then were evaluated by external reviewers who verified that the innovations did indeed work and were improvements over the previous practices. All innovations were reviewed/evaluated, and field tested, before being introduced as standard programme practice.

The programme actively developed the capacity to capture successful innovations, rapidly disseminate them, and include them in the revised programme policy and practices. The speed with which innovations could be moved from pilot activities conducted by one fieldworker to national or global practice was remarkable. This process of encouraging innovations and rapidly disseminating them reflected the two way nature of empowerment and involvement of field staff by senior management.

Finally, this chapter will discuss how the lessons from smallpox were used by other programmes such as the Expanded Programme on Immunisation, and communicable disease surveillance and response.

Programme Perspective: Innovation and Research at Field Level as a Major Programme Focus

A WHO Director-General's report to the 22nd World Health Assembly in 1969 pointed out that the malaria programme encountered serious operational difficulties. The report stated that "the present methods of eradication, although simpler than those available before . . . are still laborious and often too expensive for the limited resources of developing countries; unless the present methodology is further simplified, global eradication, though theoretically possible, will continue to be beyond reach for many years to come."[1] The report mentioned that failure to innovate and simplify was adversely affecting the malaria eradication effort.

Malaria experts sitting in the WHO headquarters in Geneva, whose job was to coordinate the global programme, began to interfere, advising when to stop spraying and how to utilise the malaria funds, failing to leave the matter in the hands of those on

[1] P. Yekutiel, "Lessons from the Big Eradication Campaigns", *World Health Forum* 2, no. 4, 1981, 470–71.

the spot who knew about the local malaria situation. The reports of independent assessment teams, which were never independent but rather dependent on the largess of local authorities, were shelved if they did not agree with the government's own views of policies or their own epidemiological criteria, which did not correspond to those developed by WHO expert committees on malaria.[2]

Malaria fieldworkers who found that the strategies were not working as expected were discouraged from modifying the strategies and, in effect, were disempowered. This was the opposite of the situation created for smallpox eradication. Smallpox fieldworkers were given wide latitude to innovate, and were empowered and encouraged to do so.

From the outset, management of the smallpox eradication programme recognised that progress with malaria eradication had slowed because of a failure to innovate and to empower field staff. The smallpox programme wished not to repeat these failures. The WHO headquarters expected programmes to be designed locally by the national staff and their WHO counterparts working in collaboration and to evolve and change with time in the light of experience. Consequently, programmes differed greatly from country to country and from time to time.[3] Taking the opposite approach from the malaria programme, smallpox leadership thought that rigid manuals of operations intuitively made little sense given the diverse nature of national health structures. Broad goals, with provision for flexibility in achieving them, became the accepted mode.[4] Fieldworkers used this freedom to innovate and design programmes suitable for local conditions.

Given the operational strategy adopted, the WHO smallpox eradication staff in Geneva viewed as their first priority a duty to

[2] M. A. Farid, "The Malaria Programme: From Euphoria to Anarchy", *World Health Forum* 1, nos. 1 & 2, 1980, 15.

[3] F. Fenner, D. A. Henderson, I. Arita, Z. Jezek, I. D. Ladnyi, *Smallpox and its Eradication* (Geneva: World Health Organization, 1988), 1361.

[4] D. A. Henderson, "Eradication: Lessons from the Past", *Bulletin of the World Health Organization* 76, supplement 2, 1998, 18.

anticipate and be fully responsive to national programme needs and to provide all possible support to them.[5]

It was in the course of executing national programmes that the most important observations were made, as a result of which significant changes in strategy and tactics were introduced. Senior management reported that there was the belief that studies conducted during the execution of programmes could do much to elucidate the epidemiology of the disease and to benefit programme implementation. There was, moreover, the belief that the potential of the tools and methods already available could be further developed to permit the task to be achieved faster and more efficiently.[6] The fact that most research was undertaken during and in the context of the fieldwork in order to answer practical questions or to resolve apparent paradoxes provided an unusual impetus to the research effort. Moreover, the interaction of research and programme execution permitted the prompt practical application of many of the findings.[7]

The target of nil incidence of smallpox—the completion of a finite task—undoubtedly played a role in motivating staff and sustaining interest. There are few health programmes which have such a clearly definable end point. However, comparable levels of achievement, interest and morale in other programmes should be possible where specific goals are clearly identified, where progress is regularly monitored and where the programme staff are fully supported and encouraged in their efforts.[8]

Encouragement and Empowerment of Fieldworkers by the Management at all Levels

The WHO managers in India recognised the need to carefully recruit, highly motivated and loyal, special purpose personnel for the campaign. With such personnel it was possible to decentralise decision making, delegate responsibility and provide fertile grounds

[5] Fenner et al., *Smallpox and its Eradication*, 1361.

[6] Ibid., 1361–62.

[7] Ibid., 1362.

[8] Ibid., 1362.

for creative problem solving. Periodic review meetings provided the opportunity to rapidly communicate successful innovations from the most peripheral field stations to programme units throughout the entire country and to maintain enthusiasm.[9]

One commentator noted that it is generally acknowledged that the vast majority of such important innovations as recognition cards, house watchguards, the reward and containment books came from field staff, and a major role of managers is that of stimulating field staff to creatively tackle problems as they arise. An attitude of problem-oriented practical experimentation in the field, with dependable support from the centre, is a prerequisite to problem solving in many programmes.[10]

One manager who worked on smallpox eradication, and later with the successful Universal Childhood Immunisation effort of the 1980s, noted that the successful leader, and especially the successful public sector leader, is one who can persuade various trumpet players to join in harmony to support a worthy goal. This requires that the players be empowered and be given credit for their contributions. This requires, in turn, that the leader or leaders involved be more orchestra leaders—intent on the results, than themselves being trumpet-blowers. Such leadership is facilitated when the goal to be attained is easily understood, when progress is easily measurable and when the goal itself is narrow.[11] These comments, made during a keynote address at a conference on eradication, refers to several levels of "trumpet players", but the comment about empowerment also applies to smallpox fieldworkers as well.

The perspective of senior smallpox eradication programme management, and the respect given to the fieldworkers, has been summed up in the acknowledgements of the publication, *Eradication of Smallpox in India*.

[9] Larry Brilliant, *The Management of Smallpox Eradication in India* (Ann Arbor: University of Michigan Press, 1985), 139.

[10] Larry Brilliant, *The Management of Smallpox Eradication in India*, 159.

[11] R. H. Henderson, "Keynote Address", *Bulletin of the World Health Organization* 76, supplement 2, 1998, 16.

> Since 1973 many epidemiologists, both national and international, worked in the programme, living and working in the most difficult conditions and for a number of hours each week, far beyond what could reasonably be asked of them. They did this cheerfully and without complaint, making an enormous contribution to the enthusiasm and spirit which percolated down to all members of the team. A major tribute must be paid to the hard core of people at grass-roots level who did the walking from house-to-house, the never-ending questioning, the spreading of information about smallpox and, when the disease was discovered, the vaccinating, living in affected villages, giving up the comforts of their own homes to live with the smallpox patients so as to isolate them effectively. To the preventive health workers of India who worked so hard for the common goal, goes our greatest acknowledgement. They did a magnificent job and our thanks go to all of them. We cannot name them all, there are too many, but each in his own way made possible the 'public health miracle' of a smallpox-free India. [12]

Almost all smallpox fieldworkers have their own anecdotes about how they were encouraged and stimulated to contribute to the programme by management at all levels. One worker felt that he was expected by senior management to solve at least one problem every day. [13] This thinking led to many achievements, including getting emergency vehicles and supplies to Somalia in 1977 within a timeframe that was thought impossible.

I remember Dr D. A. Henderson (the Director of the global programme) asking me (a very junior fieldworker) at a meeting in Addis Abeba, Ethiopia, in 1972, how I would suggest to improve the programme in Ethiopia. Again in 1973, during a holiday before returning to Ethiopia, when visiting Dr D. A. Henderson at his WHO office in Geneva, he gave me plenty of time, putting his feet up on the desk during our discussion while asking how things could be done better. This resulted in making me feel like a most important player in the programme. Of course, later, I would realise that office work accumulated while he was talking to people, which had to be done very early in the morning or late in the evening.

[12] R. N. Basu, Z. Jezek, and N. A. Ward, *The Eradication of Smallpox from India* (New Delhi: World Health Organization, 1979), x.

[13] John Wickett, interview, Geneva, September 2007.

Time spent for encouraging junior staff had to be made up later, but paid major dividends for the eradication effort.

Even after achievement of smallpox eradication was clearly within sight, management at the WHO headquarters continued to give recognition and encouragement to the fieldworkers, establishing an 'Order of the bifurcated needle'. In 1976, the addresses of international participants in the smallpox eradication effort were traced and a letter, a certificate and a bifurcated needle bent into the shape of a zero was sent to each of them. The addresses would later be useful to write to some of the same staff inquiring whether they would be ready to travel immediately to Somalia in 1977 to help with the containment of the smallpox cases detected there. The letter stated:

> Over the past three years, it has often been suggested that some symbol of recognition for participation in the smallpox eradication programme be given. . . . Appropriate recognition of national staff has been accorded by many Governments—for international staff, the symbolic Order of the Bifurcated Needle is intended as a modest recognition of an extraordinary contribution. [14]

Strong evaluation culture throughout the programme: Assessing innovations

While field staff were encouraged to seek innovative solutions to problems, assessment and evaluation remained an integral part of the smallpox eradication effort. The programme possessed an important advantage for assessment and evaluation in that there was one key indicator—zero smallpox cases—to measure progress against. The evaluation could ask and answer the key question of whether the number of smallpox cases was decreasing. By the end of the programme there were also well developed indicators and a surveillance system which could be used to monitor the programme and detect if the innovations were improvements.

[14] Letter from Dr D. A. Henderson to the fieldworkers, Geneva, 1976 (personal files).

The importance of evaluation to the programme is highlighted by Dr D. A. Henderson in his preface to the official account of the eradication effort in India:

> The success of the campaign I feel reflects the principles of sound management—a clear identification of objectives, a definitive plan for carrying out the programme, the development of techniques for independent assessment of what was being achieved factually and modification of the programme accordingly, functional delegation of responsibilities and authority and an effective ongoing programme of staff training at all levels. Dedicated, tireless, imaginative leadership and inspired local level workers made it work.[15]

The importance of evaluation is further emphasised as one of the key components of the successes in India in several publications. Assessment—that is, concurrent evaluation—of progress towards management and epidemiological goals is an essential part of any programme. The purpose of assessment is not simply to show progress, but rather to feed information into the management information system in order to continuously change the tactics needed to meet programme goals. Assessment in the field provides supervision and encouragement to staff and creates a standard of excellence and good morale.[16] This was certainly the case for smallpox eradication.

Another India programme participant also pointed out the importance of evaluation to the successful effort.

> All the national programmes have built-in evaluation methods. The interval between occurrence of a defect/problem and its detection and the interval between the detection and correction has always been considerable. . . . In this smallpox campaign the continuous monitoring of the smallpox status, feedback from the field staff and the authority for taking on-the-spot decisions regarding fiscal, administrative and technical matters have narrowed down the unknown and unsolved problems to the minimum.[17]

[15] Basu, Jezek and Ward, *The Eradication of Smallpox from India*, viii.

[16] Brilliant, *The Management of Smallpox Eradication in India*, 161.

[17] Fenner et al., *Smallpox and its Eradication*, 789 (quoting M. Dutta et. al., "Lessons Learnt from the Intensified Campaign Against Smallpox in India

Monitoring and assessment were done at every level. The WHO epidemiologists also assessed performance of containment and searches of villages in their area. Market searches were used to check if all cases had been detected during the searches. This use of evaluation and assessment at all levels served to not only identify successful innovations, but to improve programme performance as well.

Rapid dissemination of innovations

The programme actively worked to rapidly disseminate information, particularly on innovations and problem solving. The global programme used publication of documents to record and disseminate information on innovations and research findings. The *Smallpox Eradication* series included many studies and detailed findings carried out and written by fieldworkers which would form the scientific basis for innovations put into widespread practice throughout the programme.

In the final stages of the programme in Somalia, Bangladesh and India, monthly review meetings were held at state level in India and at the national level in Bangladesh and Somalia. The meeting agendas included presentations of the current situation, problems and achievements. Internal meetings for WHO epidemiologists were also held where ideas and information on innovations tried could be exchanged. Some of the practices presented at these meetings in U.P., India, such as the four questions to evaluate the search and a smallpox rumour register, to be discussed later in more detail, would become standard programme practice.

The review meetings also provided an opportunity for WHO epidemiologists to informally exchange ideas and experiences outside of the formal meetings. The meetings presented an opportunity to share ideas, problems (misery loves company), and solutions. The meetings also allowed a chance to unwind and re-charge the batteries for another month of hard work. All WHO epidemiologists were required to attend, even if they had to drive

and their Applicability to Other National Health Programmes", *Journal of Communicable Diseases* 7, 1975, 209–13).

into the state meetings in India late in the night, after completing necessary fieldwork in the evening.

The meetings also provided an opportunity to increase camaraderie and team spirit. For example, at the U.P. state level monthly meeting in Lucknow in early 1975, during tense discussions about the discovery of outbreaks in Sitapur district, it was reported that the responsible medical officer could not be located at his Primary Health Centre. This was discouraging news just at the time everyone thought the end was near in U.P. Dr M. I. D. Sharma, Commissioner of Health and Director of the National Institute for Communicable Diseases, New Delhi, broke up the meeting in laughter by joking "Let's do a special search for the medical officer".[18] This released the tension and left people chuckling for many weeks afterwards.

Review and information meetings, similar to those in India, Bangladesh and Somalia were held in other countries as well, although the frequency needed to be adapted to local travel realities. Ethiopia had an annual review meeting during the early years of the programme, from 1972 to 1974. Monthly review meetings would have been difficult in Ethiopia as it might have taken some fieldworkers more than a week to reach to the meeting site and a similar number of days to return.

Rapid dissemination of information on innovations and implementation reflected the two way nature of empowerment and involvement of field staff by senior management. The fieldworkers were active presenters and participants at the review meetings, sharing their experiences and taking away ideas and instructions to use during the next month.

Evolution of strategies based on field innovations

One way to evaluate objectively the acceptance of field innovations and their impact on the smallpox eradication effort is by comparing the strategies at the start of the eradication programme with those at the end. Innovations, tried first by fieldworkers, were introduced

[18] Author's personal notes.

which constantly increased the efficiency and effectiveness of the programme.

It is quite remarkable that the strategies and practices at the end of the programme were almost totally changed from those at the beginning. The strategy changed from initial mass vaccination campaigns and passive surveillance to one of active searches (eventually house-to-house) and containment vaccination. At the time of the World Health Assembly resolution in 1966, mass vaccination was recommended, with countries setting goals to vaccinate the entire population in a multi-year period.

In Bangladesh, the "attack phase" from 1961 to 1963 succeeded in providing 75 million vaccinations, with an additional 68 million vaccinations recorded from 1964 to 1966. Despite the large number of vaccinations, a government review in 1965 found that the programme had achieved the result of a control programme only.[19] The existing strategy was not working.

By the end of the programme, strategies in India, Bangladesh and Somalia had changed. Active surveillance, including house-to-house searches, market searches and school searches, replaced passive surveillance. Rewards for reporting a previously unknown smallpox outbreak were offered to further improve the quality of surveillance. These innovative strategies were often developed by fieldworkers. House-to-house containment vaccination, using government workers and temporary-hire vaccinators from local communities, increased coverage in the outbreak areas. Houseguards and quarantine were introduced to stop spread of infection, again pioneered by fieldworkers.

Freeze dried vaccine was introduced, delivered using the bifurcated needle, which increased vaccination efficacy, reduced vaccine consumption by 75 per cent and made vaccination much easier to teach to community volunteers. While the vaccine and bifurcated needle were developed at global level, they were field tested and introduced in field trials in many countries, by fieldworkers.

[19] A. K. Joarder, D. Tarantola and J. Tulloch, *The Eradication of Smallpox from Bangladesh* (New Delhi: World Health Organization, South-East Asia Regional Office, 1980), 22.

Smallpox eradication programme management, recognising the errors of the centralised, inflexible malaria eradication programme, set out to create the opposite and succeeded.

Personal Perspective

Characteristics of fieldworkers

D. A. Henderson notes that in total there were about 765 individuals from 73 different countries who worked for the smallpox eradication programme as international WHO staff or as consultants. In addition, as many as 150,000 national workers were involved in the programme in the mid-1970s.[20] These numbers reflect the greatly increased operations in the last remaining endemic countries in the mid-1970s, and there were far fewer field-workers involved in the programme before this time. Even the higher numbers are rather small when compared to the number of endemic countries involved in the eradication effort and the scope of operations. These numbers also may not represent the total number of fieldworkers involved in the programme if one considers also non-health staff such as government leaders, community leaders and members, private sector workers mobilised by their companies, religious leaders, teachers, students, drivers, interpreters and others, who also made important contributions to the success of the programme.

The involvement of non-health staff can be seen as another successful aspect of the eradication effort. The programme's ability to motivate and involve many people outside the health sector in its vision of a world free of smallpox played an important part in the success. While some were paid for their involvement in the programme, like temporary vaccinators or hired house guards, others were not, and many supported the programme without any financial reward, or in ways out of proportion to the payments they received. Fieldworkers, both international and national, allocated considerable amounts of their time to educate people about the purpose of the eradication effort and the feasibility of getting rid

[20] D. A. Henderson, *Smallpox, The Death of a Disease: The Inside Story of Eradicating a Worldwide Killer* (Amherst, New York: Prometheus Books, 2009), 104.

of the disease. Education sessions were held in governors' offices, schools, tea shops and, in Ethiopia, in ordinary houses in villages where teams discussed the purpose of their visit long into the night while drinking coffee around a fire before sleeping overnight in the village. Education was also helped by knowledge about the reward for reporting a case of smallpox, introduced at the end of the programme. The smallpox reward was found to be among the most widely known information at village level in some smallpox endemic countries. This is not surprising since searchers were going house to house in every village telling each household about the reward for reporting a case of smallpox. While knowledge of the reward by itself would not be sufficient to obtain collaboration, it provided an opening to discuss other aspects of the programme.

Dedicated, hard working and flexible. There were many medical officers and infectious disease epidemiologists mobilised for the eradication efforts. But in addition, the involvement of international persons like myself, who did not have medical degrees and were not necessarily initially experts in epidemiology or disease control, was an important factor in the success of the programme. These people became fully committed to the smallpox eradication effort, and worked tirelessly to achieve zero cases.

Lower level and mid-level national staff were, in turn, fully involved in the programme by WHO epidemiologists, with their ideas included in discussions and problem-solving. Often the knowledgeable paramedical assistant (PMA) or medical officer and international epidemiologist working as a team could accomplish things that each of them individually could not. Every international staff I have talked to acknowledges that no matter how hard working and motivated they were, there were several national staff with them who worked even harder and longer hours. Involving and empowering mid-level technicians, to harness their knowledge, hard work and problem-solving skills to the smallpox eradication effort, was crucial to success. Figure 5.1. shows Mr Mohammed Koodus, a member of a smallpox surveillance team in southern Bangladesh, visiting a household to investigate a suspected smallpox case.

Fieldworkers were expected to spend most of their time in the field, talking to people, educating them, and learning how the work was actually being done. The role of WHO staff assigned to the countries differed from one country to another. The most effective staff were those who served as working counterparts and took an active role in field operations. Those who assumed the more traditional role of passive technical advisers and rarely travelled outside the capital city were encouraged to leave the programme.[21]

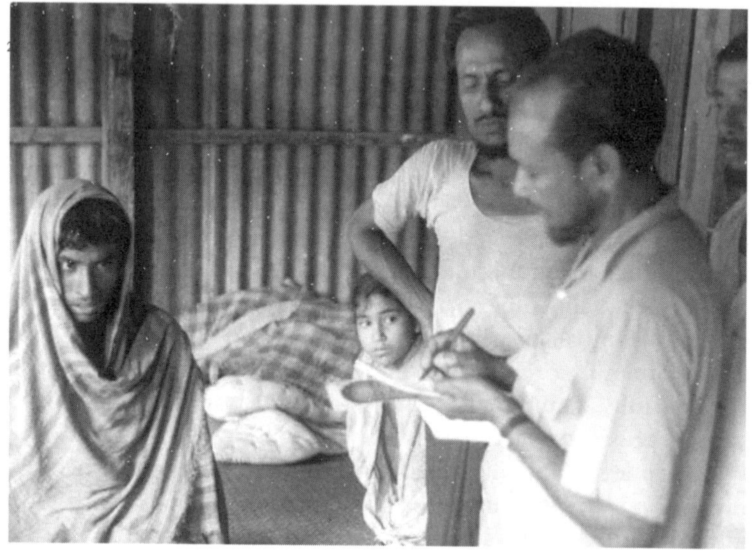

FIGURE 5.1: Mr Mohammed Koodus investigating a suspected smallpox case in Bangladesh, 1976.

Source: Photograph provided by the author.

I was reassigned from southwest Ethiopia to U.P., India, after gaining experience in surveillance and containment, and the confidence that the strategies had worked to eradicate the disease in Welega province of Ethiopia. Many other experienced Ethiopia smallpox workers also worked in India, Bangladesh and Somalia. This exchange of experiences was actively promoted by senior management. As working counterparts, WHO staff with prior experience in other smallpox eradication programmes transmitted confidence in the feasibility of eradication and were better able to introduce new methods.[22]

Optimistic. International fieldworkers were overwhelmingly optimistic that smallpox would be eradicated. Despite all the physical deprivations, there was a constant atmosphere of optimism. The fieldworkers I came in contact with never seriously thought about failure. Of course, there were many occasions when things were not going well. There were failures in containment when the work did not go as planned, when staff did not perform as expected or as they reported. But overall, from my own experience, when the work was done correctly, whether in Ethiopia, India or Bangladesh, the strategies worked. The virus disappeared.

Of course, from time to time I had doubts about whether we could eradicate this disease. One of those times was in U.P., in the winter of 1974–75, where the district I was working in (Kheri) recently had thirteen outbreaks, the most of any district in the state at the time. We had been able to quickly contain and close most of the outbreaks, but still had some active outbreaks on the books when a new one was discovered in January 1975. We used to send in a weekly aerogramme to the state headquarters (in addition to the aerogramme sent to the National Smallpox Eradication Programme office in Delhi). In these aerogrammes we wrote about the existing outbreaks at the end of the week—the new ones found, the ones closed after successful containment and the number of outbreaks pending. There was a space in the aerogrammes to request for any support required. Once after reporting the new outbreak, I wrote a comment that we needed rain to shut down the roads in order to prevent the movement of people in and out of the infected village. I asked the state headquarters in Lucknow to please send us rain. It rained several days later, after the aerogramme would have had time to reach Lucknow. The rain greatly reduced local travel and we could then easily contain the outbreak. It was then that I realised that we would certainly succeed in eradicating this disease.

Diverse backgrounds. Fieldworkers came from almost all levels of education and segments of society. Houseguards and temporary

[22] Ibid.

vaccinators were recruited from among villagers, some of them illiterate. Vaccinators were often primary or middle school graduates. Supervisory staff usually had college or medical degrees. All of these people, with their different perceptions, cultures, levels of understanding and ways of working, had to be fully involved and committed to the programme. It is quite amazing that this could be successfully done. Perhaps the success of integrating all these fieldworkers into a successful team reflects on the clear goals and simple strategy, refined and applied locally, and the good mid-level management which could translate the high level policies into understandable, doable and practical, successfully implemented activities. The successful bridging of programme efforts from highly skilled senior managers to basic health staff by the mid-level manager field staff is another clear achievement of the programme.

I remember sitting at a monthly meeting in Somalia in 1978 and reflecting on the number of nationalities represented among the fieldworkers who were sitting in randomly selected seats around the conference table: there were about fourteen persons from eight countries (Somalia, Czechoslovakia, France, Indonesia, Egypt, US, Pakistan and UK). This seemed like quite a normal situation at the time.

In Ethiopia, India and Bangladesh, international smallpox staff came from a large number of countries from both sides of the 'iron curtain'. In Bangladesh, epidemiologists and other programme participants came from twenti-nine countries, including erstwhile USSR, US, Brazil, Austria, Indonesia, France, the Netherlands, Sweden, Australia, Czechoslovakia, Egypt, Poland, UK, Switzerland, Japan, Germany, India, Bangladesh, Thailand, Philippines and Ethiopia.[23] The mix of nationalities got along well together, speaking the same language (smallpox) and sharing the same ideology (smallpox eradication). Given the environment of the cold war at the time, it was quite remarkable. The main factors affecting any disputes between people were due to someone not being fully involved in the programme and not working as hard as expected for a smallpox fieldworker.

[23] Joarder et al., *The Eradication of Smallpox from Bangladesh*, 208.

Achieving beyond expectations. Fieldworkers were encouraged at all levels to achieve beyond their capacities. This was quite remarkable in an environment, particularly at lower levels, where many workers in other programmes, may be colleagues of the smallpox eradication workers, were receiving their salaries for incomplete or falsified work, or even no work at all. One expects that this was on the mind of temporary searchers as they walked in the mud or hot sun house to house over several days. Work deficiencies happened in smallpox eradication also, but eventually through mechanisms such as use of solid indicators, constant interaction, monitoring and field supervision, the smallpox eradication programme was able to marginalise the poor work so that it did not interfere with the final success.

Each international field staff will have his or her own examples of staff who worked with them and made major contributions to the eradication effort. I will recount one of my favourites, in which I learned a valuable lesson in team work from one temporary vaccinator in India who was part of a large team of around twenty-five persons to conduct containment vaccination and search around one of the last outbreaks in Kheri district, U.P., in January 1975. A not very educated or skilled vaccinator was provided to us by an influential person and recruited against my better judgement. I did not object too much as I understood that we had sufficient capable staff to cover for an inadequate one. However, this fieldworker in the end played a crucial role in the successful outcome of the containment. Through his attempts to do his best, despite errors and tribulations, he kept the rest of the team in good spirits for the entire time. People chuckled for many weeks even after the containment was concluded. Once this worker silently and mysteriously disappeared from the back door of a jeep which was driving on a bumpy dirt road. He was found sitting on the road (unharmed), fifty metres behind the jeep, when someone eventually noticed he was missing. The group dynamics for this team were excellent, with high quality of work and cooperation. I have to think that this temporary vaccinator, whom I initially did not see the value of including in the team, played an important part.

Underachievers didn't last long

Of course, not all fieldworkers were hard-working, idealistic team players. As with any large group of people, all types and personalities were present. Some examples include:

During a containment operation in Kheri, one vaccinator received a telegram advising him "*mata bimar hai, jeldee ah*" thus informing the vaccinator that his mother was sick and he should return home immediately. However, after ascertaining that his home was quite some distance away, it was noted that the telegram originated from the post office in the next village. His request for leave was refused!

A major disagreement with an international supervisor in Ethiopia occurred when he did not see the benefits of involving national colleagues from other programmes in the smallpox work. Despite having a very capable and interested national colleague in the provincial health office, the supervisor actively discouraged this person from getting involved in the programme, countering my efforts to get him involved. After heated discussions with Addis Abeba headquarters, this supervisor was reassigned.

On another occasion, a newly arrived international short term consultant was taken on a field trip to introduce him to the smallpox eradication work. He talked a lot about the very nice lifestyle of WHO consultants, who stayed at nice hotels and did not do strenuous work. He expected the same in Bangladesh. But the speedboat he was travelling in was caught in a small canal at low tide, after taking longer than expected to check some rumours, as the water level decreased to levels where the speedboat motor could not work. Attempts were made to push the speedboat through the water and mud to a larger canal, although without success. This consultant was not accustomed to this type of work and preferred to watch from the bank of the canal. The water eventually completely drained from the canal and we had to wait for the water to rise again. The consultant was rather discouraged by this type of dirty and manual labour and he left after one month, without completing his contract. International epidemiologists who expected to have comfortable living conditions, and only intellectual type of work, did not last long as fieldworkers in the smallpox eradication programme.

Work: Composition and Workload

From challenging to mundane work

Daily work was varied, ranging from the challenging to the mundane. And one never knew what the day would bring. Anything was possible. A searcher might report a new smallpox outbreak, or someone at a teashop would inform about a case of smallpox sending us off in unexpected directions. The work was often challenging: when planning search programmes, convincing people to get vaccinated, defusing confrontations between staff and villagers or convincing governors to support the programme. It could be extremely interesting at times, like when doing epidemiological tracing of the source of an outbreak, organising containment teams or establishing containment programmes. Of course, there were also routine activities which needed to be done like training programmes for searchers, paying per diem to workers, fixing the vehicle, although even these routine activities could quickly escalate into the category of challenging work if the workers presented too many falsified receipts, or rebelled as a group because their per diem was too low, or repair of the vehicle entailed tense explanations to the driver and repair shop that the speedometer/odometer cable (used to monitor the petrol consumption) should never break, and if it broke again the driver would be fired or transferred. And of course, there were the mundane activities, with no chance of moving to other categories like preparing reports, doing accounts and completing forms and other paperwork.

Overwork and stress

The workload was always heavy and there were never enough hours in the day to do all the necessary tasks. Some fieldworkers used to work eighteen hours a day and then sleep while driving between outbreaks late at night. Fieldworkers remained in the field for about twenty-six days a month (at least), working at least fourteen hour a day (and often more), doing strenuous work such as walking house to house, walking or bicycling between villages. Rest was taken during meetings at the provincial/state or national capital or upon returning home between field visits. This was a time to catch up on activities such as writing reports, cleaning clothes, taking hot showers/baths, reading mails, catching up on international newspapers, exchanging stories, experiences and advice with other smallpox workers, and generally recharging batteries.

Stress levels varied by country and stage of the programme, but were usually high. There were always difficult management decisions to be made about organising and supervising large teams, defusing conflicts or interacting with local staff who may not yet have fully understood the programme, often under time pressure, without all the facts, and while tired.

Differential diagnoses of smallpox cases in particular raised the adrenaline. When local staff were in doubt about the differential diagnosis, international epidemiologists were expected to provide confirmation of whether the case was smallpox, with the need to immediately decide whether to start containment or not. Laboratory results were not available for several weeks. A challenge vaccination (used to help distinguish between severe chickenpox cases and smallpox) would take several days for a result. Decisions needed to be made quickly and accurately.

Normally, differential diagnoses were easy. But in some cases, it was very difficult to differentiate. Differential diagnosis and the decision to start containment were much easier at the start of the programme, when there were many cases. At the end, when any missed case was potentially the start of new outbreaks, it became more difficult. The question 'does this look like smallpox?' was easier than 'are you 100 per cent sure that this is NOT smallpox?' Often in adult chickenpox (the disease is more severe in adults), it could be difficult to differentiate from smallpox in the very early stages of the rash. All pocks could be at the same stage (like smallpox), the adult patient could be very sick including fever before onset of the rash and in bed at the time of visit (smallpox patients were normally very sick, and if the patient with a rash was walking around and had to be called back to the house for checking, the case was likely not to be active smallpox). In severe chickenpox, the rash could be present on the extremities as well as the trunk. These were the most stressful decisions, which got more difficult as the time from the last case increased.

Working environment

Living conditions were often primitive, with few amenities. In Ethiopia, fieldworkers often slept in people's houses in the villages as there were no hotels. Some workers brought tents with them on field trips. Sleeping in people's houses provided benefits of being able to talk and explain the programme in the evening, although there were also disadvantages like fleas and lice, and sharing the empty space in the centre of the mud hut with animals. It was always amazing to me that many times people in the villages stayed up quite late at night, talking by the light of a small wick lamp. At times I had to excuse myself, after starting to doze off, saying I needed to sleep. My assumption that village people went to sleep when the sun went down proved to be incorrect.

For outbreaks in the last stages of the programme in Bangladesh, including the last *Variola major* outbreak in Kuralia village, Bhola, we normally made camp in the village where the case occurred. I stayed for one week in a house in Kuralia village, with other members of the containment team before being replaced by other international epidemiologists. However, I cannot say that we slept there as we were usually up well into the night doing night vaccination with hurricane lamps to catch people who had been out in the fields or boats during the day.

"Average" working day. There really was no such thing as a routine workday when smallpox outbreaks were ongoing. The work varied tremendously from day to day, between countries, and even within countries. For example, in Bangladesh travel might be by a four wheel drive vehicle in northern districts like Sylhet, while in the far south there were few large roads and travel was almost exclusively by boat, motorcycle and rickshaw. Walking often included crossing scary and shaky bamboo bridges high over canals, designed for much lighter people than international WHO epidemiologists. In India travel was normally by jeep, but could also include bullock carts, elephants or on foot, depending on the condition of the roads

and the season. Jeep travel often included frustrating waits for long periods at level train crossings while rushing to check a rumour.

In Ethiopia, travel often meant multi-day journeys in Landrovers over unpaved roads or trails that became quagmires during the rainy season. The Landrover journey would be followed by travel by mule or on foot to reach villages. Amharic has the term "*mado*", which translates literally as "over that hill", which was frequently used to describe where a smallpox case was occurring. Unfortunately, the term does not include a sense of over how many hills, so the village could be over one hill or many hills. For Ethiopian highlanders, used to walking rapidly for many hours a day, the term "close by" could mean an eight hour walk. The seasons also affected travel substantially in Ethiopia, with much time spent digging the vehicles out of mud in the rainy season. Trying to walk during the rainy season in areas with red clay which clung to boots in two kilogram clumps was challenging. A trip which might be a fifteen minute drive in the dry season could become a two hour slog during the rainy season.

Examples of activities

Some examples of the field activities undertaken during the smallpox eradication work in Ethiopia, India, Bangladesh and Somalia are given below to illustrate the range of activities undertaken. The great variation between each of these countries can be noted, which demonstrates that smallpox eradication programmes were not uniform, but tailored for each country, although centered on the same basic foundation of smallpox surveillance and containment.

Activities varied markedly between the different stages of eradication. At the beginning stages, when there were many smallpox outbreaks per epidemiologist, the main focus was on management and supervision of others to get the work done as well as possible, with little time to spend in one place. In India, in 1973, one epidemiologist might have responsibility for a hundred or more outbreaks. The time available to concentrate on each outbreak was extremely limited. At the end of the programme in India in late 1974, an international epidemiologist often covered one district, with responsibility for ten or less outbreaks. As the number of outbreaks came down to a number which could be supervised more easily by one person, it was possible to concentrate on the few remaining outbreaks and ensure the quality of each one. There was more time for hands-on activities as well as management and supervision.

Surveillance and containment activities were done in all countries. For example rumours were reported from many sources which needed to be investigated, but the time and effort to investigate each rumour varied tremendously between countries. Containment vaccination might entail going house to house in an urban area, or walking for eight hours in sparsely populated countryside to vaccinate a dozen houses. During containment supervision, it was essential to check house by house in an infected village to ensure that no one was missed. This process was repeated when closing an outbreak, to ensure that there were no remaining cases.

Market searches were key sources of information in all countries. People, often coming from many villages, would assemble in the market, and those travelling long distances would provide information about a large area. Faces were also checked for scars, as experienced smallpox workers could quite accurately estimate how long ago a case had occurred, based on the status of pockmarks. Recognition cards were shown to people when inquiring if they knew of any current smallpox cases or those which had occurred in the last two or three months. Vaccination scars could also be checked to get some idea about the vaccination coverage in the area. Education about the smallpox eradication effort could also be provided to people attending the market. One of the first things to do on arrival in an area to conduct surveillance, or on discovering a new outbreak, was to identify the nearby markets and market days to utilise them for surveillance and vaccination. My notebooks contain many lists of markets and their market days, and also the results of interviews during the market search.

School searches were also important sources of information. The students were bright, interested and aware of what was going on in their villages. In some secondary schools, students would be requested to check for smallpox cases in their villages over the weekend and report back to the teachers. The teachers were

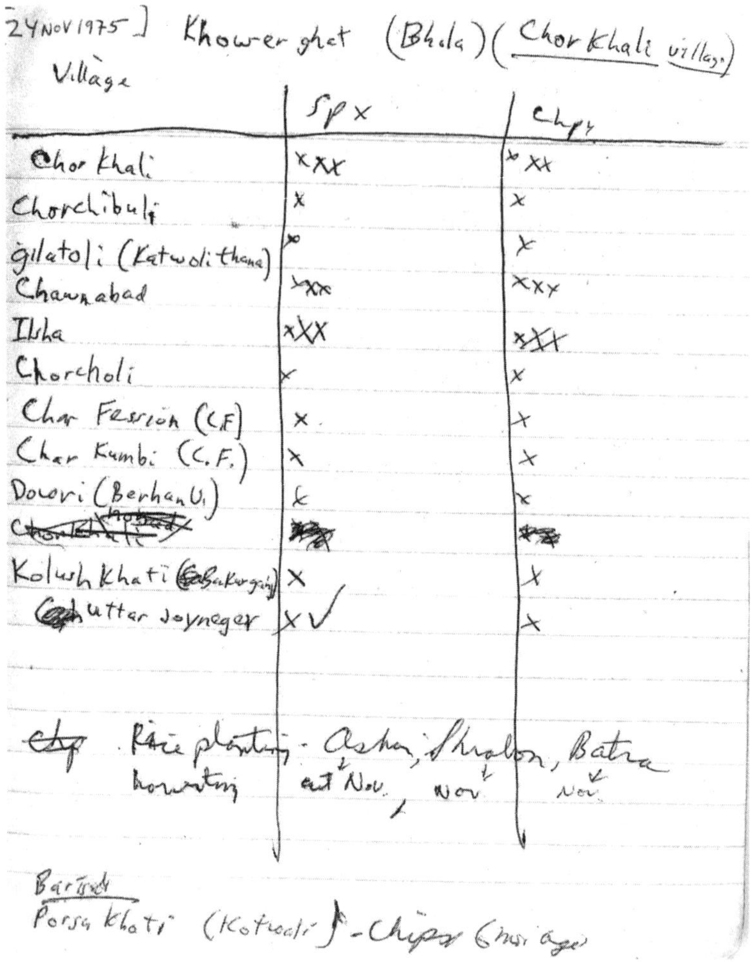

24 NOV 1975] Khower ghat (Bhola) (Chor Khali village)

Village	Spx	Chpx
Chor Khali	xxx	xxx
Chorchibuli	x	x
gilatoli (Katwoli thana)	x	x
Chawnabad	xxx	xxx
Ilsha	xxx	xxx
Chorcholi	x	x
Char Fession (C.F.)	x	x
Char Kumbi (C.F.)	x	x
Dowri (Berhan U.)	x	x
Kolush Khati (Bakerganj)	x	x
Uttar Joynegar	x ✓	x

Rice planting - Ashon, Shrabon, Batra
harvesting at Nov., Nov, Nov

Barisal
Porsa Khati (Kotwali) - Chipx 6 mos ago

FIGURE: 5.2: A page from the author's notebook shows the results of a market search for smallpox and chickenpox cases during the containment work around the last case of *Variola major* smallpox (and the last case of smallpox in Asia) in Koralia village, Bangladesh. An "X" indicates someone reported the absence of disease in a village while a tick mark (✓) indicates the presence of disease. The page shows a report of smallpox in Uttar Joynagar, which was already known.

Source: Copy of a page from the author's notebook.

also important sources of support and information, particularly in remote rural areas. The last outbreak in Kheri district in U.P. in 1975 was found through a search by school students.

In all the countries, international epidemiologists worked with the local health workers as much as possible. While the number of health workers in Ethiopia was limited, they were kept informed of smallpox activities and provided support by delivering supplies, or following up on issues, whenever possible. In Bangladesh, the counterpart was often the sub-divisional medical officer of health. In U.P., at the district level, international epidemiologists worked closely with the deputy chief medical officer (health) (DCMO(H)), or the chief medical officer (CMO).

In India, international epidemiologists had no authority to take any action except to report back to the senior district health staff, so the power to influence events depended on the relationship with the DCMO(H) or the CMO. In the case of a good relationship, lower level staff understood that reports of the international epidemiologist would be seriously considered by their supervisor and that they needed to cooperate. Senior district health staff had the power to transfer staff to a less favourable location, or at least make a recommendation that staff be transferred, which was an important consideration for lower level staff. There might be issues between the block medical officers and senior district staff, so it did not always follow that everyone seriously cooperated, but without the support of the DCMO(H), the results would have been much less successful. Of course, the interest of the district staff in the programme was affected by many factors, including pressure and perceived priority of senior staff at state level. The international epidemiologist also could write to officials at state level, although this could adversely affect the relationship with the district staff. In Kheri district, I found that most of the block (Primary Health Centre) medical officers were cooperative, ranging from very involved and spending much of their time at outbreaks to ordering their staff to pay close attention. Of course, there were a few, usually more senior medical officers, who were not interested in field issues, but in the final stages of eradication in late 1974 there were few enough outbreaks that district smallpox staff could be focused on these problematic blocks to get the necessary work done.

Government leaders at all levels were contacted in all countries. The foreigner-national team could often get access to senior officials which nationals alone could not. The programme or containment operation was explained, and support requested. Normally, the village leaders in an area would be contacted before the start of containment, to inform them and request their support. The work went much more quickly and successfully with the support of the village leaders.

In all countries, there was always much data to be reviewed and analysed, usually in the evening or late at night. The days were reserved for supervising workers and visiting villages. Data which needed to be analysed included search results by thana (Bangladesh) or Primary Health Centre/block (India) to look for gaps or unbelievable data; vaccination coverage data; assessment reports; and accounts submitted by searchers/vaccinators and surveillance teams.

In India and Bangladesh, periodic, systematic house-to-house searches were organised. These required a lot of time for preparation, implementation, supervision and analysis of results. Normally training sessions would be held to brief staff and review plans to ensure that no villages were left out and there was just the right amount of staff who would receive WHO per diem (not too many or not too few). Copies of search schedules were maintained so that concurrent supervision could be carried out to locate staff (and supervisors) in the field. After the search, house to house visits were made to review the quality of the work of the searchers, with the number and proportion of adequately searched villages calculated.

An example of an activity conducted during a search in India was to validate the searcher complaints that it was not possible to cover the number of houses assigned per day in a sandy area along the river bank on the border between two districts. The block medical officer and the WHO epidemiologist then borrowed bicycles and carried out a house to house search in the sandy areas to better understand the workload and exactly how much time was required. The assessment showed that it was fully possible to cover the expected number of houses within one working day, which was duly informed to the workers.

International epidemiologists often paid the WHO per diems directly to government staff assigned as searchers and vaccinators following a search or containment operation so that there would not be any local intermediaries, who might take a commission. While there was no guarantee that workers would not anyway have to provide a small payment to those who helped them to get the work, direct payments increased transparency. The payment sessions also provided an opportunity to discuss directly with workers the quality of their work found during assessments. This might entail praise or criticism depending on the quality of work. In the case of excellent work it would include a bonus, paid for out of pocket by the WHO epidemiologist since there were no provisions for reimbursement of this type of expense.

Some Anecdotes

On many occasions in India, I would visit the Primary Health Center at block level (covering a population of about 100,000 at that time) and meet with the medical officer. For the initial visit there was often a long presentation of how well the work was being done, followed by lunch, which took longer than expected to arrive. After lunch, the Primary Health Centre staff would then wish us a good trip back to the district capital which had more comfortable guest house or hotel accommodations where they assumed my team and I would be staying. The medical officers were often surprised to learn that, actually, we were not going back to the district capital but were intending to stay the night at the block, either in a rather basic government rest house (*dak bungalow*) or else by putting our bedding on one of the desks in the Primary Health Centre. We would then take the medical officer with us the next morning to visit a sample of villages to see if they were visited as reported. It was often quite a surprise for the medical officer in some villages as we went to house after house and interviewed villagers who all said that they had not seen a vaccinator or searcher in their village in many years, or that the searcher had visited the village, written in red chalk (*geeru*) a slogan about the smallpox reward on one of the walls and then left without talking to anyone. After a few episodes of Primary Health Centre medical officers being taken along for these types of visits to villages, the work tended to improve.

It took a bit of time to establish rapport with the drivers and other field staff, but once done, it improved the working atmosphere and the work. In India, on taking my jeep from U.P. state headquarters on my first visit to Kheri district where I was to work, I followed a practice, established in Ethiopia, of getting an estimate of the vehicle petrol consumption so that one had a better idea of when to break a busy schedule to buy petrol. I did this by filling the tank just before departure from Lucknow and again immediately after arrival at the district capital in Lakhimpur-Kheri after driving about 200 km. Later on, when the fuel consumption was found to remarkably decline, even though the vehicle was driving on asphalt roads and not using four wheel drive, this could lead to a discussion with the driver about the importance of not having to worry about running out of fuel. A weekly subsidy from my personal funds ended any problems with loss of fuel. On another occasion, on the first field trip, the driver refused to drive over a rather small ferry across a canal to investigate a smallpox rumour, saying the ferry was not safe and the vehicle would fall into the water. After checking with people, I then drove the vehicle on and off the ferry, both going and returning. That was the last time that this was necessary and afterwards the driver's performance improved and we got along well.

International fieldworkers depended heavily on their drivers, interpreters and, in India, their paramedical assistants. No matter how hard international fieldworkers worked, there were always national co-workers or counterparts who started their day earlier, accompanied the international fieldworkers, and ended their days later than them. These staff have often been acknowledged in books, articles and stories, but perhaps not enough. In each district in U.P., there were usually two paramedical assistants assigned to work on smallpox eradication. In Kheri district, Mr Iqbal A. Khan, the senior paramedical assistant, had a lot of field experience, and knew well the situation in the district. He had many ideas on how to address and resolve problems, but since he was not a medical doctor did not have much influence in the District Health Office. I was able to incorporate his ideas and suggestions and present them to the DCMO(H) as my own, which gave them a better chance to be considered and acted on. So in effect, the international fieldworkers were able to input not only their own credibility, but also involve the inputs and creativity of national staff who would have been less involved in decision making otherwise.

Abdur Gafoor, a speedboat driver in Bangladesh, was one of the dedicated smallpox eradication fieldworkers. He worked tirelessly and effectively to get our team to the places needed, often, as shown in Figure 5.3, in difficult situations. One evening while trying to return to our sub-division headquarters, we were caught in a huge area of water hyacinths in the middle of one of the branches of the Meghna river as the sun set. The speedboat propeller kept getting stopped every few seconds by the almost solid surface of water hyacinths which made progress almost impossible. As the sun set, we were caught out at night without any lights or ways to guide us to land. Gafoor persisted and eventually we saw a very dim light on the horizon and headed for it, and from there could then move along the banks of the river to find our home port. He was a totally dependable person, had a good sense of humour, eternally optimistic, and he took his work very seriously, making a major contribution to the successful eradication efforts in Bangladesh.

Settling disputes was part of the work of the WHO epidemiologist. It was not clear who was at fault in one village in India where the village pradhan (elected leader) complained that "the smallpox teams took two chickens and one egg without paying", but the dispute had to be resolved. The village pradhan also complained that the vaccinators "forced people to take vaccination and talked badly to the women".[24] After discussing this issue with the pradhan, I agreed to pay for all things taken by the vaccination teams and he agreed to accompany me to see the improved quality of the vaccination work. In another village, I was urgently called to mediate where a local villager had his *latti* (large stick using for walking and defence) raised and about to hit a vaccinator because the vaccinator had

[24] Author's personal notes.

touched his wife. As I jumped out of the jeep and walked up to the scene, the fight was about to begin. I brought my palms together, in the traditional form of greeting, and said "*namaste*" to the villager, who, as custom required, put down his latti and brought his palms together in a return "namaste". I then placed the stick to the side and we started the discussion about the cause of the problem.

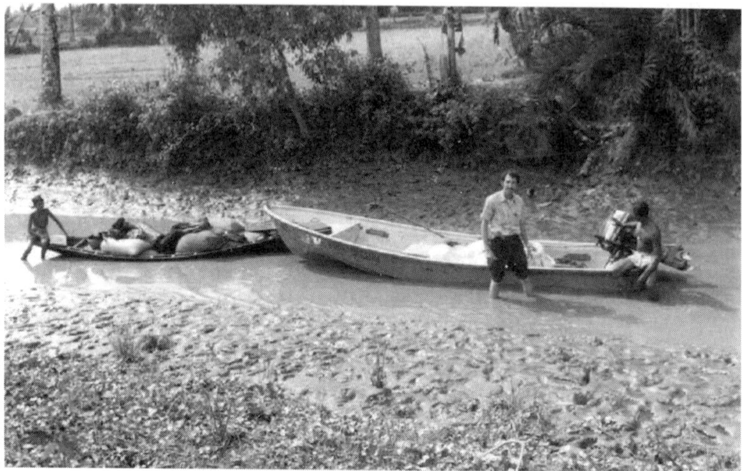

FIGURE 5.3: Travelling through canals in southern Bangladesh could turn into a race against low tide. While returning from checking some rumours, Abdul Gafoor and the author attempted, unsuccessfully, to push their speedboat to the larger canal before the water reached low tide. They finally had to wait, along with other local boats, until returning tide raised the water level.

Source: Photograph provided by the author.

The police were called into help with an outbreak in Kheri district in late 1974 only once. With some trepidation, and following mixed advice from local smallpox staff, I made a statement to the police that one person was advising people in an infected village not to take vaccination. I expected that he could be spoken to or even detained until after the containment vaccination was complete. This was the first, and last time, that I called police into an outbreak. The outcome of the police action was that a person who was helping with vaccination was arrested for illegally making alcohol, while the one who was hindering vaccination could not be found. Contrary to the findings mentioned in the article "Intimidation, Coercion and Resistance in the Final Stages of the South Asian Smallpox Eradication Campaign, 1973–75",[25] I found in late 1974 in central U.P., that it was much more effective to cultivate support from village leaders and use persuasion and persistence to get the containment vaccinations done than coercion. This was similar to examples cited in *Expunging Variola: The Control and Eradication of Smallpox in India 1947–1977*. I found the following text quoted from the smallpox programme instructions in *Expunging Variola* as correct advice: "Vaccinators should avoid tactics which frighten children. Patient, persistent effort with the assistance of village leaders will be more effective than the use of force".[26] I found from experience that intimidation did not work well as we did not actually have the power to force persons to take vaccination, and if some people were vaccinated through physical force, it would make the remaining job much more difficult as people would hide or temporarily leave the village.

At the time of the report of the last case in Kuralia village, Bangladesh, there was some unrest occurring in Dhaka, with all UN staff restricted to Dhaka and not allowed to travel. After receiving the cable about the case, Stan Foster and myself, covering our heads with light blankets to avoid detection, were driven to the ferry station to take the overnight ferry to Barisal. From there we took a speedboat across a branch of the Meghna river to Bhola island where we continued our journey by vehicle and finally on foot to the infected village. While approaching the village there was some concern whether this would be an easy or difficult diagnosis. While walking, I could see the large zero on the board at the smallpox office in Dhaka staring down at us. In the end, the case was clearly smallpox, and confirmation of the source of infection,

[25] Paul Greenough, "Intimidation, Coercion and Resistance in the Final Stages of the South Asian Smallpox Eradication Campaign, 1973–1975", *Social Science & Medicine* 41, no. 5, 1995, 633–45.

[26] Sanjoy Bhattacharya, *Expunging Variola: The Control and Eradication of Smallpox in India, 1947–1977* (Hyderabad: Orient Longman, 2006), 230–47.

search for additional cases and augmentation of the already started containment vaccination were instituted immediately.[27]

Dangerous Situations

Almost all fieldworkers have their stories about dangerous situations encountered. Several fieldworkers would pay with their lives for their dedication to achieving the smallpox eradication goal. Others would be kidnapped by guerrillas, or work every day with every possibility that they could be shot at, robbed or killed.

Flimsy eighteen-foot fibreglass speedboats were used on the large rivers in southern Bangladesh. Safety standards at the time did not require life preservers, although I am not aware of anyone who thought about this aspect at the time. The danger in this was often evident as the rivers could become quite rough, as was the case for Dr A. B. M. Kamrul Huda, sub-divisional medical officer of health, who died while travelling by boat to investigate a smallpox rumour. In another case, a speedboat sank at night, with an international epidemiologist remaining in the water for quite some time before being rescued by a passing fishing boat.

Some dedicated, and very courageous, WHO staff worked under very hazardous conditions in Ethiopian provinces bordering Somalia before and during the time the provinces were under the control of the Western Somalia Liberation Front. But their work helped to control the last outbreaks in the Ogaden, prevent any importations into Ethiopia from Somalia and provided assurance to the international community that there really were no smallpox cases occurring there.

I would not say that I was exposed to particularly dangerous situations when compared to some other fieldworkers. In fact, my experience probably fell into the "less dangerous" category. But I offer a few of my experiences as examples of "low risk" work.

In Mota awraja, Gojjam, Ethiopia, one time I was told to wait for several hours in a house by myself while my guide (Ato Asefa) discussed with the local people why I should not be robbed. Ato Asefa,

[27] Alan Schnur, "WHO Epidemiologist Tour Diary" (Dhaka: unpublished, 1975).

a well respected person from the area, but not a government official or formal leader, in addition to protecting me, was a major force for convincing people in this remote part of Gojjam to get vaccinated, which prevented spread of an outbreak from neighbouring areas.

In Somalia, while driving a Landrover with a broken clutch from Dinsoor town to Baidoa town in Bay region, we had to wait in the rain for a long time en route at a swollen river for the water to go down. As we finally approached Baidoa town, just after dark, we were confronted by an armed checkpoint outside the town, but because there was no clutch, the vehicle continued to move forward even after applying the brakes. The vehicle eventually came to a halt when the engine stalled, but the soldiers were not sure that the vehicle would stop and were aiming their guns at the driver (me) and occupants. After checking the vehicle, and on hearing that the clutch was not working, the checkpoint soldiers helped to push the vehicle so we could shift into second gear to continue the journey into town.

In Somalia, we usually slept outside of the small thatch huts on folding camp cots. After sleeping outside in one compound, we were later informed that lions had entered this compound and eaten some sheep about a week after we slept there.

Driving was always a risk. Muddy roads during the rainy season in Ethiopia often went along cliffs with a steep drop-off and no railing or protection against sliding off. In India, traffic was not well disciplined and roads were crowded and could be slippery, especially after it rained when the oil on the road came to the surface. One time, in India, we slid off the road, just missing a tree, where the jeep tipped over on its side. Fortunately, no one was injured and after we climbed out of the vehicle, people from a passing car helped us push the jeep back on its wheels again, and we drove off!

Problem-Solving as Part of Daily Work

Fieldworkers were constantly coming up against problems in their daily work that needed to be resolved or overcome. Solutions for problems were routinely being tried by fieldworkers, some elegant and others less so. Many worked, and others could be discarded after trial (such as calling the police to help with containment vaccination). But international epidemiologists recognised that any innovations and solutions needed to be culturally appropriate and suitable for local conditions if they were to have a chance of being effective over the long term.

Candies (toffees) were found to be very useful as rewards for children after they received vaccination. They also served to lighten the containment atmosphere for the adults as well as children. In India, often older children would bring their younger brothers and sisters for vaccination to get the candy for them. In one case, while a team member was trying to convince a reluctant parent to vaccinate her children, the children were already being vaccinated at the back door, with the older sister taking the candies. We did not receive any reports that this was harshly received by the parents. In one case, I wrote in my notebook at the time how an older woman was upset with me because we had run out of candies. We used to buy several two kilogram bags of hard candies per containment. Since this could not be charged to the official imprest account, it was paid for by the WHO epidemiologist. The candies were found to be culturally appropriate in India and Bangladesh and helped to speed up the containment.

In Ethiopia, there might be the need to buy a mule or donkey because a fieldworker could not easily rent one of acceptable quality for the times and places that were needed. But the regulations forbade buying any transport. So we paid for the mule, deducted the amount returned when we sold it after completing the work, and then divided the difference by the number of days worked to arrive at the daily rental fees. We could always find someone to sign this form showing how much we had paid "as rent".

In Ethiopia, adults could be reluctant to provide information, but if we could come across younger, pre-adolescent boys and girls (say about ten or eleven years old) minding the goats/sheep they would often provide useful information on smallpox cases or the location of people's houses. We began to seek out these children en route to villages if they were in a group. This was done in culturally appropriate ways, with a clear understanding that it would not have been appropriate to speak to a lone older girl in the field.

Overcoming resistance to vaccination in at least some villages in all countries proved to be a common problem. As mentioned above, in India and Bangladesh, during the later stages of the programme, it was found through experience best to involve village leaders and elders and make repeated visits to houses when necessary. Repeated visits were a powerful tool to convince people to get vaccinated, as they got the idea that the team was serious and they could not escape by putting it off. Forcing people to be vaccinated was not a viable long term solution as it only built up further resistance. In one outbreak in India among tribal villages, near the border with Nepal, after the local vaccination teams had located and vaccinated all the people accepting vaccination, it was left to the international WHO epidemiologist to study why the reported number of people vaccinated did not coincide with the reported population of the village. It was found that many people could not be located and were reported as being outside the village. In the end, a good natured room to room search of houses with flashlights, accompanied by the village leader, would detect adults and children hiding under beds, in chests, large wicker baskets and even in large clay storage vessels. However, the search was done as a game of hide and seek, with laughter after people were found and vaccinated, such as in one particular case where lifting the cover of a large wicker basket revealed two children hiding inside. It is unlikely that this containment vaccination could have been successful if people were forced to take vaccination and without the support of the village leader. It is my impression that the presence of a foreigner, who could help to turn the exercise into a game, was also important in this situation.

Every day brought new problems to solve in all categories of the work from getting support of senior officials or village leaders, to defusing conflicts between vaccinators and villagers, to winching a vehicle out of the mud when there were no trees around.

Examples of Fieldworker Innovations

Fieldworkers played an essential role in discovering many of the key innovations that revolutionised the eradication programme and, indeed, made it possible. There are many examples already published, and this section will focus on a few selected major and minor innovations, mainly ones that I experienced first-hand.

The generic process of innovation and the factors involved has been well studied and reported on. This section will not try to recover this area. But the thinking behind the innovations used in smallpox eradication is relevant and a few examples will be discussed here. The innovations discussed here were always based on fact-based reasoning, and solid analysis and evidence, and not the result of wild experiments to see what would happen. Fieldworkers, after living day after day in remote areas, and walking through villages, going house to house and speaking to local people developed a good feel for the local situation. This could be used to make a fairly accurate estimate of the effect of an innovation and its chances of success.

Arguably, the most important field innovation was the strategy of surveillance and containment vaccination which was developed during fieldwork in Nigeria, and refined by fieldworkers in countries stretching from Brazil to Indonesia. Simple devices like the bifurcated needle and plastic needle containers greatly simplified vaccination and needle sterilisation, increased efficiency and reminded us every day that the best solutions were usually the simplest ones.

Other examples are discussed below:

In Ethiopia, in 1971, the overall strategy of search and containment was fixed, but the operational tactics of stopping transmission in each province were left up to the provincial teams. At the beginning of intensified smallpox eradication activities in Welega province, western Ethiopia, large outbreaks were found, and vaccination was conducted in the centre of the outbreak area. Starting in autumn 1971, provincial smallpox teams decided to change tactics as the number of cases were too many to cover all of them with available resources. Surveillance data were analysed and the vaccination efforts moved to the fringes of the outbreak, to vaccinate in areas where the smallpox was moving, but cases had not yet occurred. An example of a vaccination session is shown in Figure 5.4. This effectively put a ring of vaccinated persons around the outbreaks to break the chain of transmission. This change in tactics contributed to a rapid decline in cases and interruption of smallpox transmission in the province. Welega in mid-1972 became the second province in Ethiopia to interrupt endemic transmission and reach zero cases, and the first province with more than one million population to do so. Although importations occurred in Welega in early 1973 (from Gojjam), they were easily contained and transmission interrupted.[28]

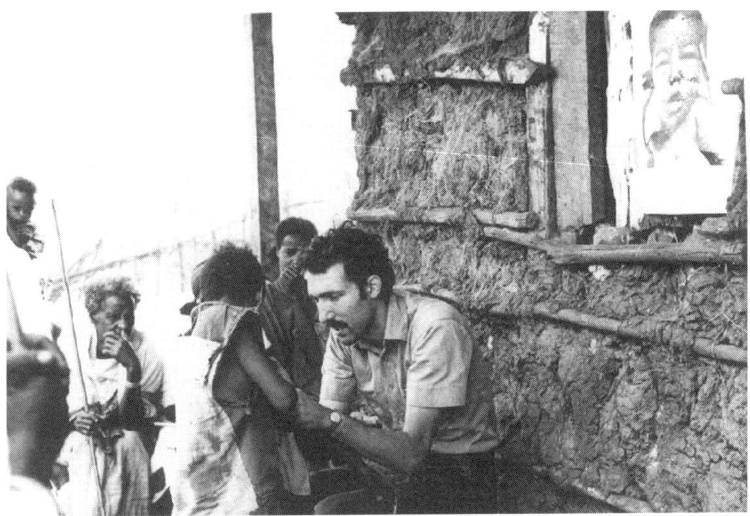

FIGURE 5.4: A smallpox vaccination session in a remote village in western Ethiopia in 1972. The smallpox surveillance and vaccination teams reached even very remote villages and were often the first government health service teams to reach these areas.

Source: Photograph provided by the author.

In U.P., in 1973 and 1974, the Government of India's National Smallpox Eradication Programme guidelines for smallpox containment required vaccinators to vaccinate all household contacts, 100 per cent of the inhabitants of the surrounding households and perform all primary vaccinations in the remainder of the affected

[28] Yemane Tekeste, Alebachew Hailu, C. do Amaral, P. R. Arbani, O. Ismail, L. N. Khodakevich and N. A. Ward, *Smallpox Eradication in Ethiopia* (Brazzaville: World Health Organization, 1984), 39, 51 and 53.

village (or *mohalla* in urban areas). Despite direct instructions from my supervisor to the contrary, in October 1974, I initiated vaccination of all people in infected villages (both primary vaccinations and revaccinations) rather than only those not previously vaccinated. This innovation was implemented based on the finding that ascertaining the vaccination status of all was time consuming and at times inaccurate. I found some old people were being exempted from vaccination because they reportedly had smallpox or were previously vaccinated. This behaviour in Indian villages was very similar to the practice of villagers in Ethiopia. In Ethiopia I found that once there were no exemptions from vaccination, the village could be covered faster as there were less discussions. In addition, in Ethiopia, once more than half the village could be vaccinated, there was a "snowball effect" with the remaining villagers coming forward for vaccination as they feared missing out on what others had already received. Similar increases in speed of vaccination and increased coverage from the "snowball effect" was also found in the villages where I worked in U.P. I understand that this strategy was also tried in parallel by others in U.P. and shown by evaluations to allow a more rapid and complete coverage of the village. After assessments showed that this revised strategy worked, it was introduced as standard practice throughout U.P. within just a few months. The term "snowball effect" was used at the U.P. monthly state review meeting when introducing the new practice. This is another example where the monthly state meetings contributed to the exchange of ideas and rapid dissemination of findings.

Introduction of house watch guards to vaccinate anyone entering an infected household was initially started by fieldworkers. This practice was tried independently by several fieldworkers in India, in one instance to keep active smallpox cases at home when there was a large fair (*mela*) near the infected houses, before it became national policy.

In India, after much field experience, four questions were standardised to assess search operations when visiting villages. These questions were: (a) if the household had been visited, (b) if the worker had shown the recognition card, (c) if the household member was told about the reward by the searcher (and knew how much) and (d) if the household member was told where to report if he should see a case of smallpox (and could demonstrate they knew where); were used previously in different variations by several WHO epidemiologists and discussed at meetings. The new assessment technique formalised and tested by Dr Walt Orenstein and Dr Don Francis was presented at the monthly U.P. state review meeting at the end of 1974. Following the presentation, the practice was standardised throughout the state, which established common indicators and allowed comparison of search quality across districts.

A smallpox rumour register was developed by Dr R. C. Johri, DCMO(H), in Kheri district, U.P., in early 1975, to immediately enter all rumours received at the district office to ensure that none were lost and also to enable monitoring of the timeliness of investigation. The rumour register was presented by the WHO epidemiologist at the U.P. monthly smallpox review meeting in Lucknow and later adopted for use throughout the state, with the title eventually changed to 'rash with fever register'.

Somalia cross border searches were developed by field epidemiologists to ensure there was no smallpox transmission in neighbouring inaccessible areas of Ethiopia. The methodology as described in the book *Smallpox and its Eradication* was ingenious, utilising signatures of local officials signed on cards which would be left by one worker and collected by another. Using multiple teams of workers to validate the work of previous teams fostered high quality work even in areas where international epidemiologists could not reach. When international epidemiologists were able to re-enter the Ogaden, they found that the work had been adequate. [29]

Containment at the last outbreak in Bangladesh in Kuralia village, Bhola sub-division, Barisal district in November 1975 was state of the art, using all the methodologies developed up to that time. The following actions were immediately taken by the international epidemiologists reaching the case to expand on the work already started by the surveillance team that had discovered the case:

[29] Fenner et al., *Smallpox and its Eradication*, 1055–56.

Teams of houseguards, including the head of the household were immediately posted at the house of Rahima Banu;

Maps were made of all villages, initially within 1 mile of the household with the smallpox case but later extended to 1– 1½ miles, showing every house, based on the readily available malaria village maps. Names of all family members were entered into registers to allow for follow-up and checking of any rash with fever cases (which could have been emerging smallpox cases);

All fever cases within the containment area were logged and followed up daily to look for any onset of rash;

The houses within 1–1½ mile radius were divided up among teams of vaccinators with every house rechecked for fever cases each day. Houses were marked with chalk for each visit and with a unique team and house number which allowed identification of the team which had visited the house and rapid identification of any missed houses;

Night time vaccinations were done using lanterns and flashlights at households and markets to catch any persons who had been out during the day, starting on the night of the day the international team members reached Kuralia;

Markets, schools and medical practitioners within five miles of the infected household were regularly visited and searched. People were interviewed at markets (and ferry stations), with the names of villages where people came from and any reports of smallpox or chickenpox noted;

Meetings of the vaccination team were held each morning and evening;

Supervision was continuous and widespread.

One innovative technique developed for the Kuralia containment effort was the highly aggressive identification, tracing and follow-up of *any* persons who had been present in the affected villages during the time of the outbreak. During the vaccination and surveillance work around the outbreak in Kuralia, workers recorded the details of any person who had visited the area during the outbreak period. Despite some initial surprise and reluctance by the radio operator in Dhaka due to the large numbers of persons who had visited during the holiday season of Ramzan and Eid (which occurred during this period), a policy of sending cross notifications by radio to other districts for all people who had been present in the infected villages during the time of the outbreaks was implemented. Since there were no other cases anywhere in Asia at the time, these persons were those at highest risk of becoming infected and continuing transmission. These persons were tracked down and checked for any evidence of rash.

Conclusions

Chipmunk effect: Fieldworkers, each in their own way, made crucial contributions to the successful effort. Mr S. Balasubramanian, a clerk in the smallpox eradication unit at the WHO Regional Office in New Delhi, who went on to play an important role as a member of the Expanded Programme on Immunisation unit, used to tell a story about how the chipmunks got their stripes after helping Rama build the bridge to Lanka to free his wife, Sita. The chipmunks were small and could not do much, but they helped to build the bridge as best as they could and to the best of their ability. In return Rama stroked their back which is how chipmunks got their distinctive stripes. The contribution of all the fieldworker "chipmunks" to smallpox eradication was substantial.

Fieldworkers were motivated and empowered to contribute to the programme and to innovate by the conscious efforts of management at all levels of the programme. Crucial innovations, contributing to the ultimate success, were made by fieldworkers in every country. These innovations were based on experience and sound knowledge of the programme conditions in the field.

Assessments and evaluations were used extensively in the programme to verify that the programme was progressing and which innovations were beneficial. The programme established a system to capture innovations and rapidly disseminate findings on successful innovations. This resulted in innovations rapidly being put into practice, within the country of innovation, or globally, as appropriate.

Lessons for other health programmes

Many of the things mentioned are well-known management principles, and are not rocket science. So maybe the greatest success of smallpox eradication was in actually applying these principles and turning them from theory into reality. Other programmes can review their own working methods and see how close they come to matching the practical application of the principles used by the smallpox eradication programme. The 'can do' practical approach and attitude of smallpox eradication carried over to other programmes, most directly to the Expanded Programme on Immunisation (EPI). The programme nominally achieved the rather ambitious Universal Childhood Immunisation goal of 1990, which was called 'a public health miracle' at the time. The leaders and many national and international EPI workers, in the WHO headquarters, in several of the WHO regional offices, and in the countries, were former smallpox eradication workers. Principles similar to smallpox eradication were followed: recruit capable country staff, support them, and, most importantly, listen to them.

The list of former smallpox eradication staff who went on to fill senior positions is long. Also notable is the list of mid-level fieldworkers who entered the programme without a health or public health background, but went on to get advanced degrees in medicine or public health and entered a public health career after the smallpox eradication programme.

Smallpox eradication also had some effect on a participant of the Severe Acute Respiratory Syndrome (SARS) outbreak in China, where I found myself remembering the smallpox eradication work while working at the WHO office in China. During the low point of SARS in early May 2003, the situation was not optimistic. The outbreak was spreading rapidly in many provinces and Beijing, with more than 100 new cases being reported every day. The streets, shopping malls and markets in Beijing were eerily deserted, with the large People's Hospital across the street from the Ministry of Health building (which shared a cafeteria with the Ministry of Health) closed down and barricaded due to SARS infections. Meetings with Ministry of Health officials to prepare workplans were held in a largely deserted cavernous Ministry of Health building. During this time, the smallpox experiences crossed my mind. There had been situations before where smallpox cases were spreading all around, seemingly out of control, and the outcome appeared in doubt. But we never doubted the outcome for smallpox, and later for SARS, since there were demonstrated successful strategies to control the disease. Just as we were sure that we would eventually reach to zero smallpox, the same single-mindedness, learning from previous successful innovations in Guangdong province to control the disease, and refusal to accept defeat also applied to the SARS work. The WHO in its discussions with the government never altered the goal from eliminating SARS as a public health threat. With such a terrible and dangerous disease there could be no question of allowing it to remain endemic, just like for smallpox.

It is well accepted that smallpox eradication worked and succeeded in large measure because of the selfless devotion of many key mid-level managers-fieldworkers. These fieldworkers were not just doing a job to see a curve go down on a graph, or to publish papers in respected journals. There was great readiness to share ideas with other fieldworkers, both informally and at meetings. This will explain why for some of the critical innovations developed at field level, it is not always possible to identify the person responsible. It was often a team effort.

For such a huge and successful undertaking, which many people initially thought as impossible, one has to consider how much of a factor was played by a "labour of love". Many of the international fieldworkers, who worked in villages for long periods of time, came to appreciate the countries they worked in and the people. With all the good and bad, daily petty frustrations and exhilarating achievements, I would propose that the quality and quantity of the work done by many fieldworkers reflected dedication, and a labour of love, as much as enlightened management.

Following this line of reasoning, maybe it is therefore fitting that the greatest beneficiaries of smallpox eradication have been the poorest people living in the poorest countries. If smallpox had not been eradicated there would still be no cases today in Sweden, US or UK as everyone would be vaccinated. Even in the wealthier sections of cities in developing countries, cases would be minimal as vaccination levels among the educated are higher. But without eradication, in the poorest areas of developing countries smallpox outbreaks would continue to periodically sweep through, scarring, blinding and killing those not vaccinated. Of course, these human aspects of the programme cannot be readily quantified and scientifically analysed, so they remain merely as my personal impressions. But the impact assessment of the smallpox eradication programme cannot be disputed. It is there for all to behold and benefit from.

6

Successful Eradication of Smallpox and the Prospect of Disease Eradication Efforts in the Twenty-First Century

Isao Arita and Miyuki Nakane

In this chapter, we discuss firstly the definition of eradication and briefly review why smallpox has so far been the only disease which was eradicated according to this definition. Some salient pictures of this eradication effort are presented. And, finally, problems and solution are discussed in order to forecast the feasibility of future eradication of certain infectious diseases, including poliomyelitis and measles.

Definition of Disease Eradication

The following definition refers to infectious diseases. Several terms such as control, elimination and eradication have been used to describe efforts to diminish the hazard of infectious disease to the human community. Control is defined as the effort to stop a dangerous disease from spreading or affecting more people: control of the common cold, for example. Elimination is stricter than control, with the aim of completely getting rid of a disease from the human community but being unable to exclude its return: for example, elimination of neonatal tetanus, as *tetanus bacillus* is always present in the soil. Eradication is the most strict term aiming at ending the circulation of the disease but also at extinction of the causative pathogen in the human community as well as in nature so that measures to prevent and treat the disease are no longer required and can be disestablished. Such a definition was extensively discussed at the Dahlem Konferenzen, Berlin, in 1997.[1]

Eradication: Permanent reduction to zero of the worldwide incidence of infection caused by a specific agent as a result of deliberate efforts; intervention measures are no longer needed.

It is important to point out that the definition of eradication implies a few strict conditions: first, it should be global, otherwise we cannot stop the preventive measures; second, the pathogen must have only human reservoirs, and not be sustainable in nature, including animals, so that an eradication strategy only needs to target humans; third, because of its global implications, a unified international effort is required, including involvement of resource-poor nations, with support for their eradication efforts. Such countries will need support to level up their eradication capabilities, although the effort may last only for a short period of time, say a year or some years. Fourth, there should be no long-term inaccessible areas, such as those affected to armed conflicts, to prevent the implementation of eradication activities.

If eradication succeeds, it is cost-effective as costly preventive measures can be stopped worldwide. If it fails, as has happened with some previous efforts, there should be contingency plans available, including an exit strategy as well as indicators for when eradication should be judged as not feasible, so that the money spent for eradication should not be wasted. In the concept of public health development, a comprehensive long-term approach, such as primary health care, is taken as a reference on the one end, with a short term eradication effort as a special unified effort focusing on a single target disease, on the other opposite end. Experience has shown, as in the failure of malaria eradication, that the success or failure of eradication often was debated from these two alternate points.

Current technology development is favourable to the eradication effort; vaccine and rapid and simple diagnostic methods would

[1] Walter R. Dowdle and Donald R. Hopkins, eds, *The Eradication of Infectious Diseases: Report of the Dahlem Workshop on the Eradication of Infectious Diseases*, Berlin, 16-22 March 1997, Dahlem Workshop Report (West Sussex: John Wiley & Sons, 1998).

be the important and practical tool both for nations with rich and poor resources. On the other hand, the recent synthetic biology advances, with its great potential benefit, is also of concern, because if certain pathogens can be synthesised with limited cost, the value of eradication, especially cessation of preventive measures, is at risk, requiring debate and action. [2]

Eradication Efforts in the Early Twentieth Century

Major eradication efforts were made for yellow fever, yaws and malaria early in the twentieth century, although all the programmes were not designed for meeting the definition as mentioned above. Yellow fever eradication was guided by the Rockefeller Foundation in the Americas in 1918 based on control of the mosquito vector, *Aedes aegypti*. Despite initial success in 1928, epidemics with unknown sources in Brazil revealed the presence of jungle yellow fever, where non-human primates are the reservoir of the yellow fever virus. With this finding, yellow fever eradication was no longer feasible.

In 1955, based on a World Health Assembly resolution, malaria eradication was started with intensive international cooperation, although Africa was not included as one of the target regions. Initial success in the Indian subcontinent as well as the Americas was based on effective vector control and surveillance. Substantial cooperation was available from bi- and multi-lateral organisations. However, resistance developed in anopheles mosquitoes against DDT (dichlorodiphenyltrichloroethane) insecticide, which made the vector control ineffective. Resistance to anti-malaria drugs also developed. Research to overcome these technical difficulties was not actively pursued among the total population living in malarious areas. Gradually, the progress slowed down, as shown in Figure 6.1. The high point of the eradication effort, in terms of protecting people, living in previously malarious areas was reached in 1965, 10 years after the inception of the programme. However, there was a gradually declining trend in programme achievements as the

[2] Eckhard Wimmer, "The Test-tube Synthesis of a Chemical called Poliovirus", *European Molecular Biology Organization Report* 7, Special Issue, 2006, S3–S9.

programme encountered technical difficulties. In the early 1970s, the World Health Organization (WHO) declared a shift from malaria eradication to a control programme.

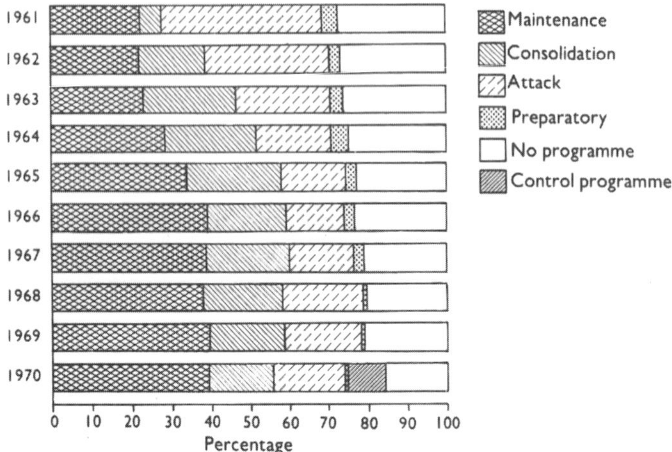

FIGURE 6.1: Percentage of population of malarious areas, by phase of campaign, 1961–70*

Note:* In 1970, the total population of the malarious areas was 1,801,631,000.

Source: R. G. Scholtens, R. L. Kaiser and A. D. Langmuir, "An Epidemiologic Examination of the Strategy of Malaria Eradication", *International Journal of Epidemiology* 1, 1972, 15–24; and WHO data.

Malaria eradication started during the period when the Second World War ended in 1945 and the United Nations (UN) with WHO were established with the aim that all the nations wished to do something good for the welfare of humankind. It is no wonder, therefore, that smallpox eradication was also discussed during World Health Assembly in 1958, three years after malaria eradication. Unfortunately, at that time, the concept and strategy for eradication was just in the initial stages. It was thought that the willingness of national governments and, if needed, provision of smallpox vaccine, would be sufficient to achieve the eradication goal. Also, in the late 1960s, when the malaria programme was encountering difficulties, as mentioned above, and when smallpox eradication was underway with slow progress, there had been no intensive international cooperation. In fact, at the WHO headquarters, the smallpox eradication programme was assisted by just one medical officer and suffered constantly from a shortage of vaccine supply. As malaria eradication successes slowed down, whether smallpox eradication should be continued was debated during a few World Health Assemblies.

Smallpox Eradication, Development and Success in Ten Years: Beginnings

In 1966, the WHO Executive Board reviewed the secretariat's report with a proposal for an "intensified" smallpox eradication programme, which described that, if smallpox eradication should succeed as planned, it should require substantial WHO regular budget to assist the programmes in the then thirty-two smallpox endemic nations in Asia, Africa and South America.[3] The proposal was based on the special report prepared by a WHO assessment team which had visited several national programmes. The proposal caused concern among Executive Board members, as the ongoing malaria eradication effort was facing the risk of failure, but the WHO secretariat was firm. Finally, after lengthy debate, the proposal was accepted by the Executive Board, which was followed by endorsement by the World Health Assembly. Accordingly, the intensified smallpox eradication programme was initiated by a newly established WHO system at the headquarters, regional and national level, and national programme offices. However, the size was much smaller than the malaria programme at that time.

The new WHO system rapidly prepared and acted on a major new strategy as detailed below.

1. A Global Commission for Eradication of Smallpox was formed to advise on programme development; it consisted of experts on smallpox, epidemiology, virology and health administration.

[3] F. Fenner, D. A. Henderson, Isao Arita, Z. Jezek and I. D. Ladnyi, *Smallpox and its Eradication* (Geneva: World Health Organization, 1988).

2. Surveillance: Surveillance was strengthened, with WHO requesting all nations to report on a weekly basis the cases of smallpox to the WHO regional offices, which transmitted the report to the headquarters. At the beginning of the programme, laboratory confirmation was not required and the reported cases were based only on clinical diagnoses. Often, reported numbers were incomplete (due to passive surveillance systems) and special active search was needed at the peripheral level or village level. Only late in 1976, when the programme was nearing the target of zero cases, the Centers for Disease Control and Prevention (CDC), Atlanta, US, and Research Institute of Viral Preparations, Moscow, in the erstwhile USSR, started to test specimens for verification of clinical diagnoses. Surveillance was sensitive due to clear manifestation of the clinical picture and further due to the fact that its speed of transmission was much less rapid than initially feared, for example as compared to influenza infection.[4]
3. Vaccine: Vaccine quality was improved, with only laboratory approved freeze-dried vaccine to be used. Under the new strategy, donated vaccine would be accepted only after testing by either of the two WHO collaborating centres for vaccine testing: National Institute of Public Health, Bilthoven, Netherlands, and Connaught Laboratory, Toronto, Canada. Freeze-dried vaccine offered greatly improved heat stability—four weeks heat stable at 37° Celsius. The final reconstituted vaccine vial was not allowed to be filled with more than 0.15 ml to 0.25 ml (ten to twenty doses with conventional scarification method) which was sufficient to vaccinate forty to eighty persons with bifurcated needles. More than this amount would cause greater wastage of vaccine at vaccination sessions at static health units or even house-to-house because the reconstituted vaccine had to be discarded at the end of the day. As the WHO regular budget

[4] R. H. Henderson and M. Yekpe, "Smallpox Transmission in Southern Dahomey: A Study of a Village Outbreak, *American Journal of Epidemiology* 90, no. 5, 1969, 423–28.

for smallpox eradication was not enough, all the vaccines had to be donated from bilateral sources.

4. Vaccination strategy and method: Vaccinations were to be done either by static health units or by mobile teams. Bifurcated needles were to be routinely used (after being donated to the programme patent-free by the US company, Wyeth Laboratories). The initial vaccination target was to cover the entire population of smallpox endemic countries within three years. Any outbreaks required immediate containment measures, including isolation of the patient, active surveillance and containment vaccination. Vaccination scars on the arm were used for verification of vaccination histories as well as assessment of vaccination coverage.

Landmark Activities

US bilateral programme for smallpox and measles eradication in West Africa (1966–73)

Around the time WHO's intensified programme started, US bilateral cooperation to eradicate smallpox and control measles in nineteen nations in West Africa was initiated in close collaboration with the WHO programme. This programme, in fact, contributed the best available technology for sound testing and development of the WHO strategy in terms of surveillance, vaccine and its administration and programme assessment. It set up a programme office at Lagos, Nigeria, and contributed about 100 professional staff from the US. The jet injector, initially the main tool used by this programme for vaccination, was five times faster than the usual vaccination method using bifurcated needles. However, later, the jet injector was given up due to frequent mechanical breakdowns. The programme succeeded in interrupting transmission, with the last case in Nigeria in 1970, within four years from its initiation. The programme's achievements greatly contributed to WHO programmes, because the operational areas contained nations with limited resources, which posed serious difficulties for the global effort in terms of operation and assessment.

Initial promotion of programme development

In 1967, as the programme in West Africa was under way, the WHO sent missions to all the endemic nations in the Indian subcontinent, Middle East and South America to initiate national programmes. The missions discussed the programme with national staff and offered transport, vaccines and operational advice as well. Thus, almost all endemic nations were able to start the programme within a year of the World Health Assembly resolution. This was not an overly difficult achievement but an important move to meet the requirement that any global infectious disease eradication programme must start simultaneously on a global scale to limit to a minimum importations from non-operational nations to operational nations or vice versa. The smallpox eradication efforts contrasted with one of the serious problems of the current polio eradication effort which has been its difficulty to start intensified efforts simultaneously and to maintain the same pace of progress in all geographical areas.

Assurance of vaccine quality

In 1967, when the programme started, the quality of vaccine in use was investigated by contacting forty-five manufacturers. Only sixteen were found to meet WHO vaccine standards of potency and stability. It became an urgent programme priority to improve this situation. In 1968, a seminar was held to prepare a manual to improve vaccine quality, and the two WHO collaborating centres—Global Centre, Netherlands and Regional Centre (Americas), Canada—were designated. They assisted national manufacturers needing improvement. The manual was sent to all the manufacturers. An arrangement was made for these two centres to test samples from every production batch. Only batches with satisfactory results were used in the eradication programme. It is noteworthy that within three years, the rate of satisfactory batches increased from 30 per cent to 80 per cent (Table 6.1).

TABLE 6.1: WHO quality control of freeze-dried vaccine

Year	*Number of producers*	*Number of batches submitted*	*Number satisfactory (%)*
1967	20	74	27 (36)
1968	23	136	74 (54)
1969	30	164	128 (78)
1970	27	380	312 (82)
1971	32	206	154 (75)
1972	27	311	241 (77)
1973	30	392	367 (94)
1974	28	231	199 (86)
1975	21	167	139 (83)
1976	16	213	203 (95)
1977	11	114	101 (89)
1978	9	59	57 (97)
1979	10	85	82 (96)
1980	5	46	46 (100)
Total	—	2,578	2,130 (82.6)

Source: Isao Arita, "Standardization of Smallpox Vaccines and the Eradication Programme: A WHO Perspective", in *A Celebration of 50 Years of Progress in Biological Standardization and Control at WHO*, ed. F. Brown, E. Griffiths, F. Horaud, G. C. Schild, Development in Biological Standardization 100 (Geneva: World Helath Organization, 1999), 31–37.

Selected National Programme Activities

In 1967, when the intensified eradication effort started, smallpox was endemic in thirty-two nations, located on three continents, with only a few nations with imported cases. After six years, in 1973, smallpox remained endemic in only six nations, with four nations reporting importations. By 1976, the disease was restricted to only three nations in the Horn of Africa (maps 6.1, 6.2 and 6.3).

South and South-East Asia

Afghanistan. Unlike today's war-torn nation, Afghanistan has a relatively developed health services. Smallpox was endemic, with cases also imported from Pakistan. Transmission was interrupted in 1973, with the last case which was an importation from Pakistan. Variolation was practiced, with the smallpox crusts stored for long periods of time in the cold weather conditions found in the

MAP 6.1: Countries reporting smallpox case in 1967

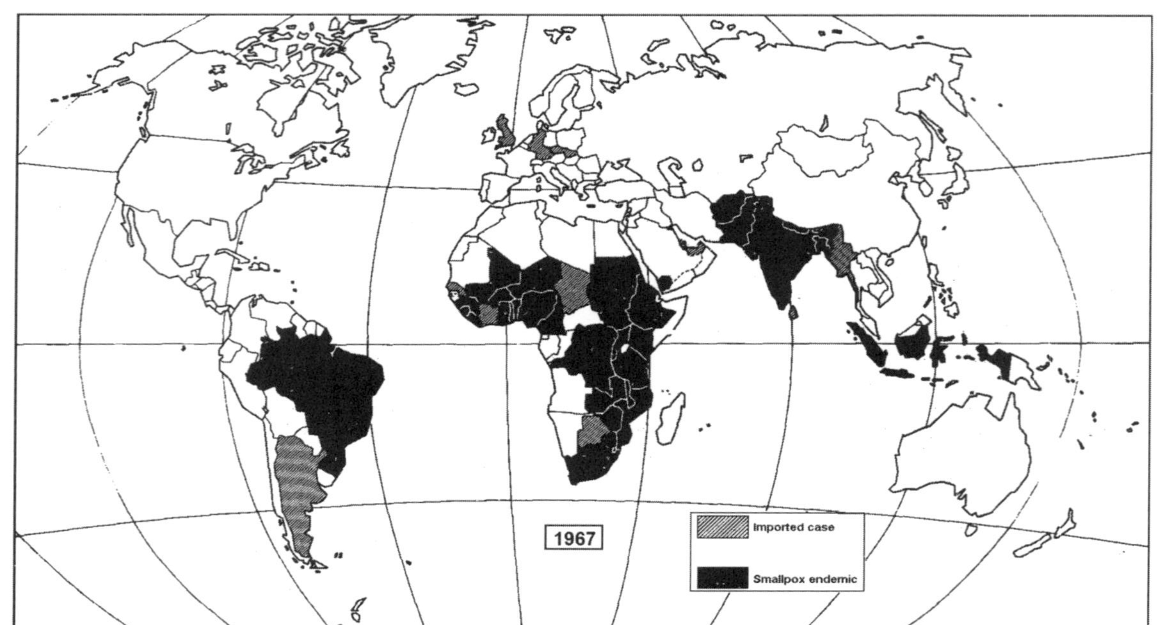

Source: World Health Organization, *The Global Eradiation of Smallpox: Final Report of the Global Commission for the Certification of Smallpox Eradiation* (Geneva: World Health Organization, 1980).

Map 6.2: Countries reporting smallpox case in 1973

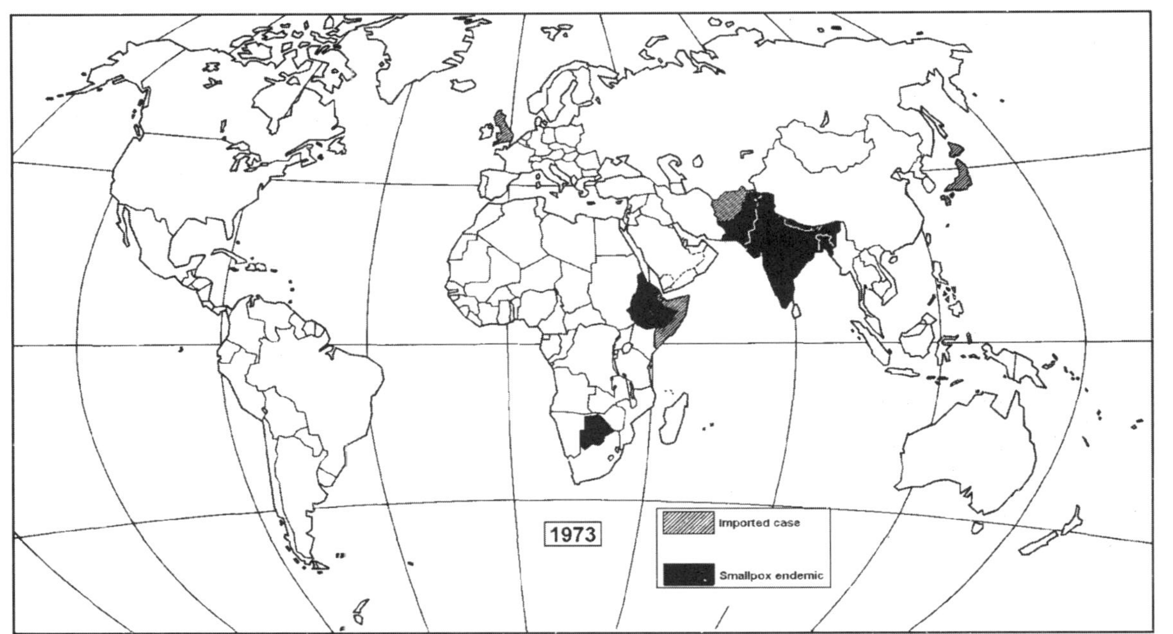

Source: World Health Organization, *The Global Eradiation of Smallpox: Final Report of the Global Commission for the Certification of Smallpox Eradiation* (Geneva: World Health Organization, 1980).

Map 6.3: Countries reporting smallpox case in 1976

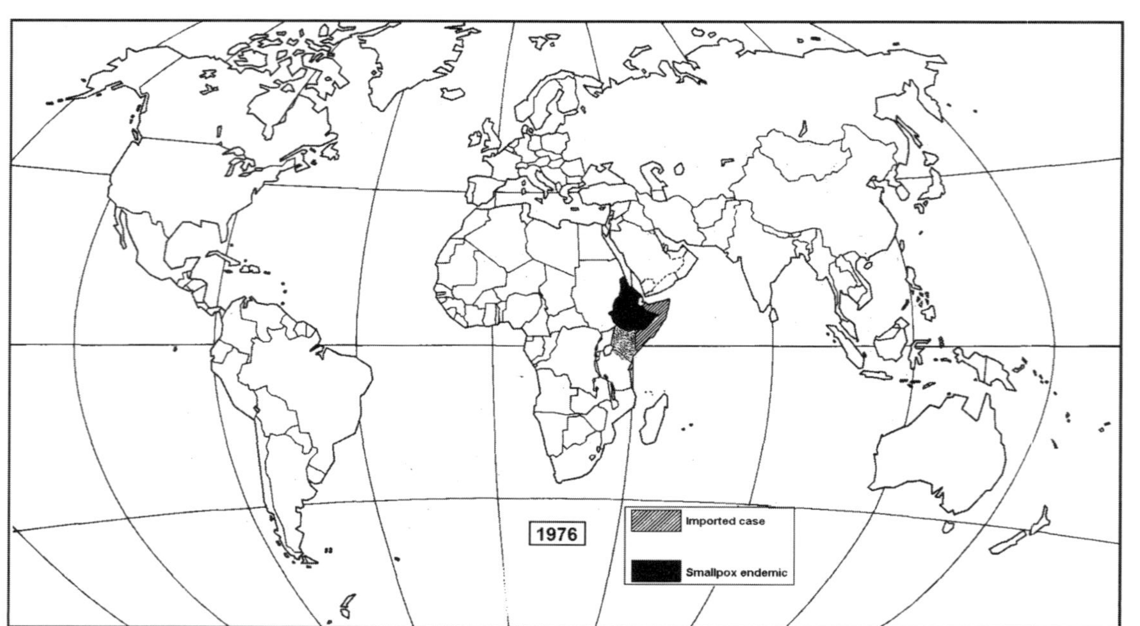

Source: World Health Organization, *The Global Eradiation of Smallpox: Final Report of the Global Commission for the Certification of Smallpox Eradiation* (Geneva: World Health Organization, 1980).

mountains. Smallpox eradication efforts succeeded in persuading the villagers or variolators to destroy their smallpox variolation specimens. Some years later, a study indicated that the stored variolation specimens were negative for virus isolation and the risk of disease return from this source was considered to be minimal.

Bangladesh. The high density of the population alongside the Ganga required extremely high vaccination coverage, which was hard to maintain. The systematic, well-organised vaccination campaigns, continuing since 1967, were not able to interrupt transmission. In 1967, however, surveillance reports indicated that smallpox outbreaks were occurring only in a belt in the northern zone. There were no reports of cases in the south. Also, 1969 appeared to be the lowest incidence year from the viewpoint of the cyclic pattern of smallpox in Bangladesh. A decision was made to stop the systematic mass campaign and to shift programme personnel to the northern outbreak zone for special active surveillance and containment of detected smallpox outbreaks. The result was remarkable. The containment project started sometime in mid-1969. About 1,500 cases occurred up to August 1970, but thereafter, no cases were detected until spring 1971, despite active surveillance to detect cases. Why only up to spring 1971? Because the Indo-Pakistan war started and in Bangladesh (then East Pakistan) surveillance teams were unable to work from April to the end of 1971 because of dangerous conditions. The programme was temporarily discontinued.

In 1972, Bangladesh reported 10,754 cases when the refugees who left Bangladesh in 1971 returned from West Bengal, India, where many had been infected by smallpox. The infected refugees, returning after the cease fire, became the source of new smallpox outbreaks nationwide. The incidence increased to 32,711 cases in 1973. This is an example of how war can influence the fate of eradication efforts in a nation. Intense efforts continued after peace was restored, using the surveillance and containment strategy, with Bangladesh reporting the last smallpox case in southern Asia in 1975, with the date of onset of rash being 16 October 1975.

India. India had started a nationwide vaccination campaign already early in the 1960s, even before the WHO intensified smallpox eradication effort was launched in 1967. However, disease incidence continued, without a distinct declining trend. A cyclic pattern of epidemics was noted. Surveillance was not sensitive, leaving continuing hidden transmission. Meanwhile, several smallpox endemic nations with a large population had become smallpox free: Nigeria in 1970, Brazil in 1971 and Indonesia in 1972. When the delayed eradication effort caused concern among the international community, in consultation with WHO, the Indian health services prepared a drastic strategy to complete the programme. In 1973, all health centres started to release staff for one week in every month for surveillance/containment actions. The teams visited every village first to search for smallpox cases and then to vaccinate fifty households surrounding the case detected. The case was isolated in a nearby house with a guard. If no further cases occurred for six weeks, the village would be removed from the list of infected villages. This system was meticulously carried out by the teams with participation of WHO consultants. The project termed "autumn campaign" resulted in remarkable success. It started in September 1973 and ended in May 1975, with the last smallpox case in India. Notably, during the campaign, with improved surveillance, the incidence soared up to 188,003 cases in 1974 from 88,003 in 1973. These figures indicated that only a small portion of cases were reported every year before the campaign (Figure 6.2). This rapid decline in cases was one of the remarkable examples of success in the history of smallpox eradication. The incidence in India in 1974 represented 86 per cent of the global total of that time. While smallpox had perhaps cause suffering and public health disasters in India from time immemorial, it could be eliminated in eighteen months with well planned and implemented special human efforts.

Indonesia. The campaign started in June 1968, with the last case recorded in January 1972. The programme provided interesting experiences for the global programme, namely instituting active searches for "unvaccinated" campaigns during which smallpox cases were frequently encountered. The success in Indonesia led to the adoption of the strategy of active search and containment vaccination at global level. This strategy of surveillance and containment, was applied in the above mentioned Indian autumn campaign. Another new technique was the use of a photograph of a smallpox patient during active searches for cases. The technique was effective, which led to the production of a "WHO Smallpox Recognition Card" (Figure 6.3). The cards were produced by the WHO in millions of copies for use by every field worker during searches for cases.

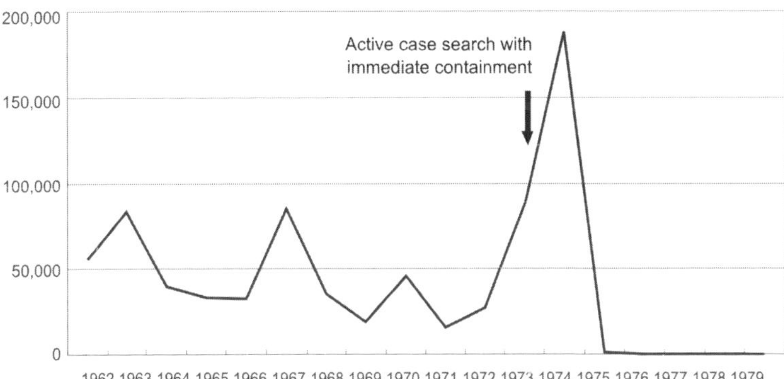

FIGURE 6.2: Number of smallpox cases reported by year: India.

Source: © World Health Organization.

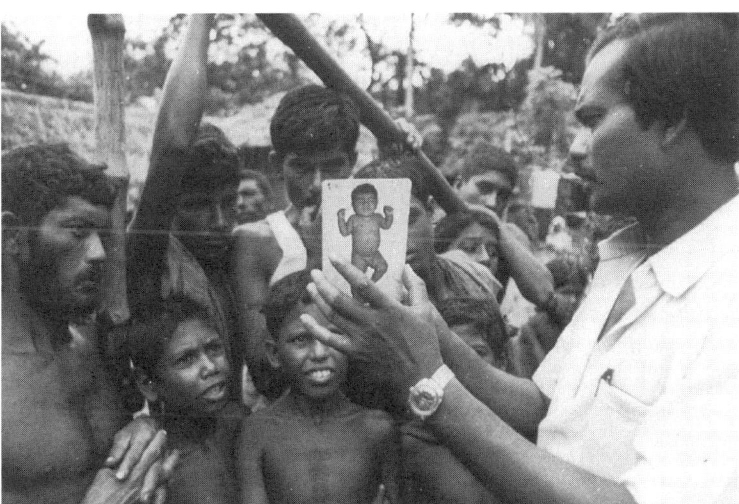

FIGURE 6.3: Active search of cases by using the smallpox recognition card.

Source: © World Health Organization.

South America

The programme made good progress under the guidance of the WHO Regional Office for the Americas.

Brazil. Brazil with its large population and vast geographical area was the major smallpox endemic nation in South America in the 1960s. The systematic vaccination programme was strengthened as was surveillance and containment work. Several thousand reporting units were established and special surveillance and containment teams formed to support the surveillance and containment strategy. Brazil recorded the last smallpox case in the Western hemisphere in 1971.

Horn of Africa

As shown in maps 6.1, 6.2 and 6.3, by 1976, smallpox transmission was circumscribed in the Horn of Africa. Hidden transmission (imported from Ethiopia) was found in Somalia early in 1977. The hidden transmission caused an importation into Kenya, which alarmed the world as at the time there had been no reports of smallpox throughout the world for a month. Emergency action was taken by the WHO. In addition to the recruitment of twenty Somali staff, twenty WHO consultants were deployed to Somalia from their stations in India, Ethiopia and elsewhere, where they were engaged in certification work after achieving zero cases. A total of sixteen Landrovers were airlifted to Mogadishu, the capital of Somalia, courtesy of the Danish military service. Rewards were offered to those who reported smallpox cases. National emergency vaccination teams were set up. All these actions were implemented within a month. Also, following telephone requests for funding in May 1977, US$465,000 was donated by the UK, Norway, the Netherlands, Canada, Sweden and International Red Cross within one month. The containment work started in March 1977, with the last case discovered at Merca, a small town in the south of Somalia, in October 1977, eight months later. This case was the last case of naturally occurring smallpox anywhere in the world, up to now. The date of onset of the rash was 26 October 1977 (Figure 6.4).

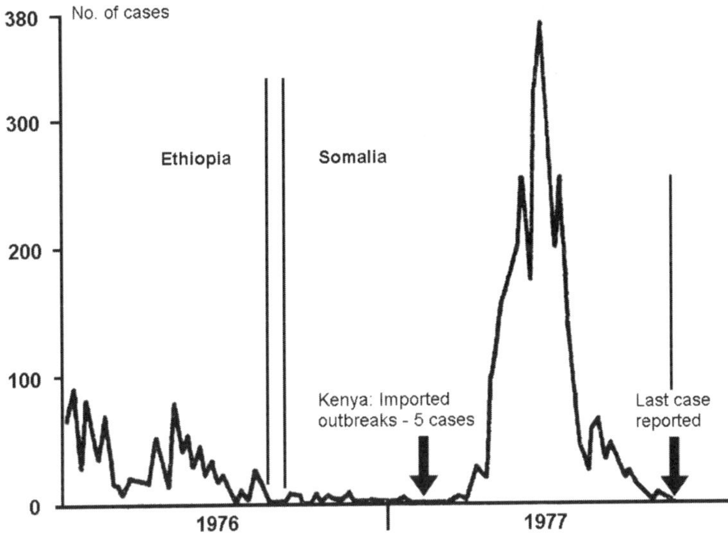

FIGURE 6.4: Weekly incidences of smallpox in Ethiopia, Kenya and Somalia.

Source: © World Health Organization.

Research and Innovation

Smallpox has a long history and was well studied before the eradication effort. However, during field operations, studies were organised with the aim of increasing programme efficiency, and several important findings were made, as described below.

Disease epidemiology

The transmission pattern of smallpox was studied in a small village, in the erstwhile Dahomey, now Benin. It revealed that smallpox spread is slow, and close contact with a case is required for infection. This finding appears simple, but it presented a sound basis for surveillance-containment as the main strategy in smallpox eradication.[3] Monkeypox virus infects humans, resulting in a smallpox-like illness, but fortunately, field studies showed that person-to-person transmission is difficult. It therefore does not constitute a risk to eradication by being a natural reservoir of smallpox-like disease. The main epidemiological studies on monkeypox were conducted in the Democratic Republic of Congo and elsewhere.[5] Efforts were made to find out serological evidence of smallpox infection with attempts to differentiate antibodies caused by smallpox virus and vaccinia virus. The studies were not successful. It was found that pockmarks appear in 80 per cent of smallpox cases, which provided the scientific foundation for the reliability of pockmark surveys.

Vaccine and vaccination

Studies showed that vaccine stocks could be increased by four times, with satisfactory take rate, by using a bifurcated needle (with fifteen punctures) as compared with the usual scarification method (unpublished data, WHO). In addition, the standard heat stability test for freeze-dried vaccine, which normally takes four weeks at 37 ° Celsius, could be shortened to one hour with one hour boiling test, by studying the correlation of vaccine titre decline in both temperature setups. This made to decrease the time needed for vaccine delivery.

Operations

Vaccination coverage needs to be routinely assessed and should take into consideration the density of the population vaccinated. The more dense the population, the more difficult to interrupt transmission.[6] This explains why eradication progress was slower in India than in less populated nations in Africa. Smallpox transmission can even die out by itself in areas with very low population density. On the other hand, densely populated areas can sustain transmission since even high vaccination coverage still leaves large numbers

[5] Z. Ježek and F. Fenner, *Human Monkeypox* (Basel: Karger, 1988).

[6] I. Arita, J. Wickett, F. Fenner, "Impact of Population Density on Immunization Programmes", *Journal of Hygiene* 96, 1986, 459–66.

unvaccinated. Laboratory results are normally quite accurate, but it is possible to make an incorrect diagnosis, possibly related to inadvertent contamination with smallpox virus in the laboratory. While this is rare, surveillance officers needed to be careful when the laboratory result was unexpectedly different than the clinical or epidemiological observation, as happened several times during the smallpox eradication programme. When cases were too many, it was found that just recording the number of cases in each village, and the names of villages where outbreaks were occurring, was often sufficient to conduct containment operations. This saved field workers' time and labour for recording names and other data and allowed field workers to concentrate on containment vaccination. This was, in fact, the instruction by the WHO to field staff in certain field conditions.

Certification

With the last case of smallpox discovered in Somalia, in October 1977, the programme entered the phase of certification, namely to verify whether the case in Somalia was really the last case globally. If this could be confirmed, all the nations throughout the world could disestablish all control measures for smallpox, following the definition of eradication. Needless to say, the certification criteria should be technically and financially sound, so that it would be accepted by all countries.

The principle established for certification was that all smallpox endemic countries had to continue surveillance and vaccination programmes for two years after the occurrence of the last case. In addition, it was decided that countries sharing borders with the endemic countries, and also any nations without solid surveillance data, should be included in the system for certification. The method for certification included a visit by a certification team, a pockmark survey of young people in the population born after the last case, review of the smallpox rumour register and whether the reward for reporting of smallpox cases had been publicised, as well as examination of available programme records (Figure 6.5).

REWARD · RECOMPENSE
$1000
Smallpox Variole ОСПА Viruela Smittkoppor
The World Health Organization offers US $ 1000 to the first person reporting an active smallpox case resulting from human-to-human transmission and confirmed by laboratory tests. Valid until global eradication is certified.
L'Organisation mondiale de la Santé offre une récompense de US $ 1000 à la première personne qui signalera un cas actif de variole résultant d'une transmission d'un être humain à un autre et confirmé en laboratoire. Cette offre est valable jusqu'à la certification de l'éradication mondiale.
天花 चेचक Furuqa Ndui

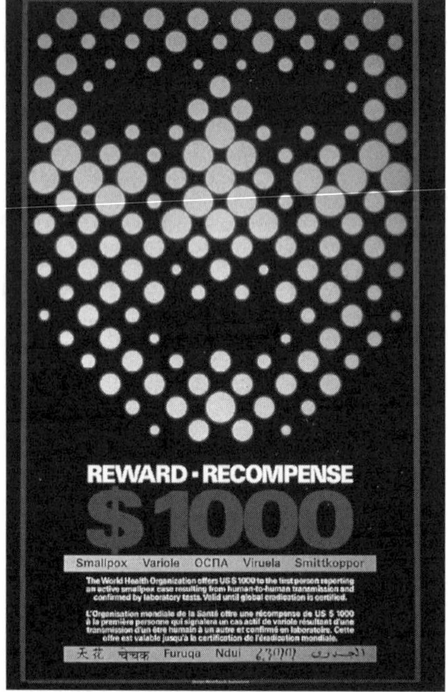

FIGURE 6.5: Reward for reporting of smallpox case.

Source: © World Health Organization.

Certification of the transfer or destruction of all laboratory smallpox virus specimens was given special attention through communication with all countries. Official confirmation of nil specimens from ministers of health in all nations was required, and, if needed, visits of teams to laboratories having reported smallpox research over the last three decades were made.

The WHO set up smallpox collaborating centres at Atlanta (US) and Moscow (former USSR), so that those laboratories who did not wish to destroy their virus strains could transfer them to these two laboratories which both had certified high security levels. The tragedy of a laboratory associated smallpox outbreak in UK in 1978, offered an opportunity to accelerate this procedure to assure the destruction or transfer of viruses maintained in laboratories. The timeline for certification activities, by country, is shown in Figure 6.6.

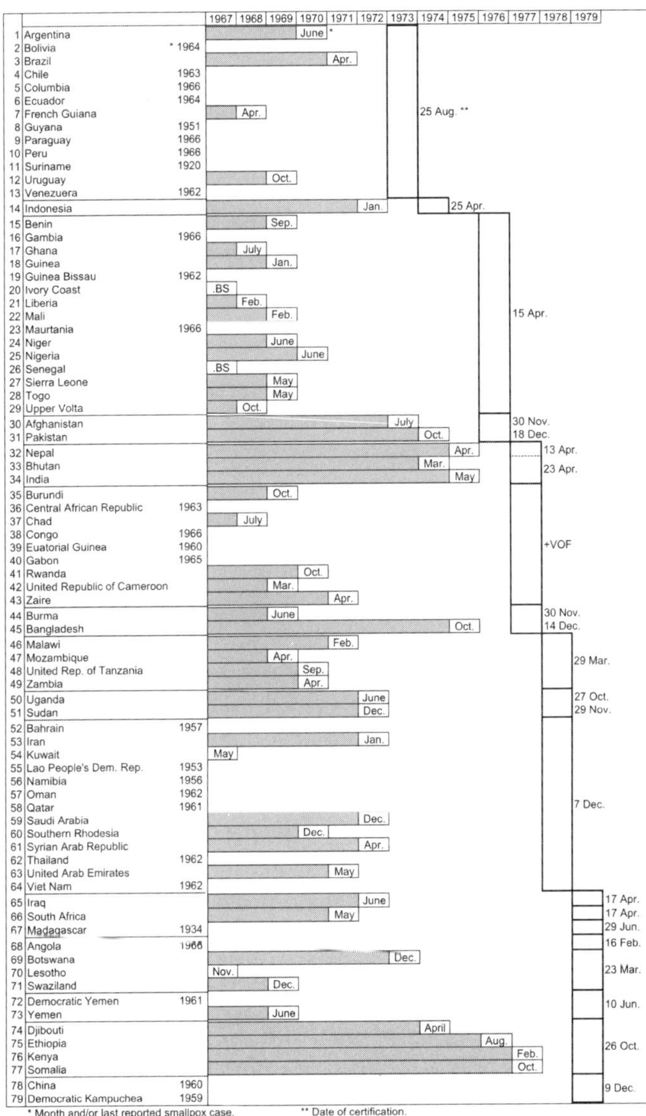

FIGURE 6.6: Seventy-nine countries which required special procedures for the certification of smallpox eradiation showing month of last reported smallpox case and date of certification.

Source: World Health Organization, *The Global Eradication of Smallpox* (Geneva: World Health Organization, 1980), 58.

In May 1980, World Health Assembly approved the report of the Global Commission for the Certification of Smallpox Eradication and declared:

> The world and all its peoples have won freedom from smallpox, which was a most devastating disease sweeping in epidemic form through many countries since earliest times, leaving death, blindness and disfigurement in its wake, and which only a decade ago was rampant in Africa, Asia and South America.[7]

Aftermath of Smallpox Eradication Success

Influence of smallpox eradication success on health services development

The success of smallpox eradication influenced the area of health services development in two ways: first, to consider targeting another disease for eradication and second, it led to more comprehensive overall consideration of health service development. The first outcome can be regarded as a logical development because the successful eradication effort provided enormous benefit to the global community in terms of disappearance of misery as well as financial saving, which was estimated as an annual saving of US$1 billion in global health costs as compared to only a total of US$300 million spent for the ten-year intensified global programme.

As for the second outcome, the eradication effort aimed at only a single target disease, and this often caused concern among health administrators, who wanted more efficient horizontal programmes to make the best use of the limited health resource available. During the failing period of the malaria eradication programme in the 1970s, the concept of primary health care and strengthening basic health service was getting more and more support, which provides a good example of the second outcome. Smallpox eradication succeeded, but the second outcome still appealed to the major groups in the international public health community.

[7] World Health Organization, *The Global Eradication of Smallpox: The Final Report of the Global Commission for the Certification of Smallpox Eradication* (Geneva: World Health Organization, 1980).

As a middle path between a vertical eradication programme and horizontal programmes came the development of the Expanded Programme of Immunisation (EPI), which was successfully developed after smallpox eradication and still continues. The EPI aims, as part of the primary health care, at strengthening of immunisation programmes worldwide with available vaccines, such as DPT (diphtheria-pertussis-tetanus), polio, measles, hepatitis B, Hib (Hemophilus influenzae type b), etc. Starting from very low coverage of 20–30 per cent in the 1970s, many nations in Africa and Asia have dramatically improved their immunisation coverage with these vaccines as a result of the successful EPI efforts. In 2005, the World Health Assembly, considering the successes achieved so far, further endorsed EPI's Global Immunisation Vision and Strategy (GIVS), which, in addition to EPI, promotes actively to introduce as many new vaccine as available and to integrate EPI with other health programmes as practical.

Prospects for eradication of other diseases in the twenty-first century

As previously mentioned, the success of smallpox eradication revealed that there should be the following three conditions for successful global eradication:

1. There is no animal reservoir,
2. the pathogen does not have recurrent infection after a period of time (such as herpes virus infection) and
3. The availability of technical tools to interrupt transmission which are effective both in rich and poor nations.

Polio and measles both meet these three conditions and when the intensified EPI efforts started to show some reduction of these diseases, plans to eradicate them were considered by the international community, first in the region of the Americas.

Americas. It is interesting to note that the concept of disease eradication appeared with yellow fever eradication in the Americas early in the twentieth century, well before malaria eradication was targeted in mid-century. Even consideration of measles eradication can be traced back to the 1960s in the US. Thus, the scientific community in the Americas, has shown a remarkable interest in disease eradication, which might be related to their pioneer spirit, as represented by the Rockefeller Foundation's sponsorship of yellow fever control/eradication efforts in Cuba and Panama early in the last century.

It was thus not surprising that after the success of smallpox eradication, the Pan American Health Organisation (PAHO) and WHO Regional Office for the Americas reviewed the reduction of polio incidence due to the good performance of EPI and decided to launch a polio eradication programme on a regional basis in 1985. Three years later, the programme was followed by a World Health Assembly resolution in 1988 to launch an effort for the global eradication of polio, with the target of zero cases by the year 2000.

Global Polio Eradication

The initial polio eradication strategy was developed by PAHO. The strategy includes four principal components:

1. High vaccine coverage is to be achieved with Oral Poliovirus Vaccine-Sabin strain (OPV)—the vaccine of choice. This vaccine can develop intestinal immunity in vaccinees and also infect contacts through the faecal-oral route. This is a great advantage as the unvaccinated may get the vaccine virus infection and be protected although they have not been given vaccine themselves.
2. Surveillance for cases of acute flaccid paralysis (AFP) is established as a means of detecting all cases of poliomyelitis, even if misdiagnosed. Faecal specimens are taken from all AFP cases and sent under refrigeration to designated laboratories for poliovirus isolation. Any poliovirus isolated is further tested for characterisation of wild or vaccine (Sabin) virus. AFP is caused by several causes, including polio and Guillain-Barre syndrome and, as experience has shown, the usual ratio is one AFP case per 100,000 population up to fifteen years of age. Establishment of an indicator for AFP

surveillance enabled it to serve as a good index as to whether surveillance for children with acute paralysis is sensitive.

3. Vaccination method is to vaccinate the entire population under five years of age (predominant age group affected by polio) during winter time, the time of lowest frequency of the polio transmission. The ease of oral administration of OPV, which allows mobilisation of non-physicians to provide vaccine, is a good advantage for vaccination campaigns.

The programme in the Americas was successful, with the last case of polio in the Americas occurring in Peru in 1991, six years after initiation of the polio eradication efforts. After considering the reports from continuing surveillance, the Regional Certification Commission for the Americas in 1994 certified that the case in Peru was the last endemic polio case in the Americas (Figure 6.7).

Eradication programmes also started in the other five WHO regions (Europe, the Western Pacific, the Eastern Mediterranean, South-East Asia and Africa) around 1990 (except Africa, which started in the mid-1990s). The other regions employed the same strategies as mentioned above for PAHO. Following the successful campaign by PAHO, the Regional Office for the Western Pacific (WPRO) succeeded in stopping transmission in the region with the last case reported from Cambodia in 1997. The region was certified as polio free by the Regional Certification Commission in 2000.

However, following certification of the interruption of endemic transmission in the European region in 2002, progress became slower. The global programme missed the target year of 2000 with cases still occurring in the remaining three regions. As of 2006, there were still sixteen nations reporting wild poliovirus cases in Sub-Saharan Africa and South Asia (Map 6.4).

In early 2007, WHO held a meeting to renew the global efforts by focusing on the four remaining polio endemic nations: Nigeria, Afghanistan, Pakistan and India, with a target to stop transmission before the end of 2008.

Considering the reasons for the delays mentioned above, it is suggested that there are technical difficulties, such as the large number of polio sub-clinical infections (200 for each paralysis case) which prevent effective surveillance/containment measures as

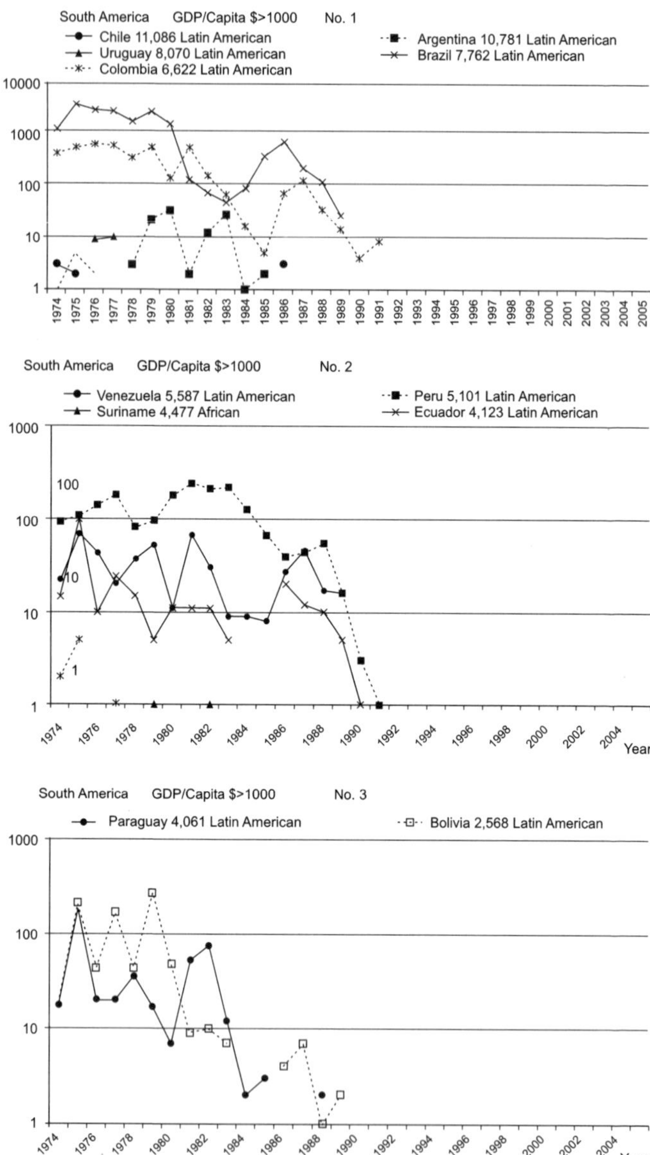

FIGURE 6.7: Progress of polio eradication in the Americas.

Source: Pan American Health Organization.

MAP 6.4: Wild poliovirus*, 21 March 2006–20 March 2007

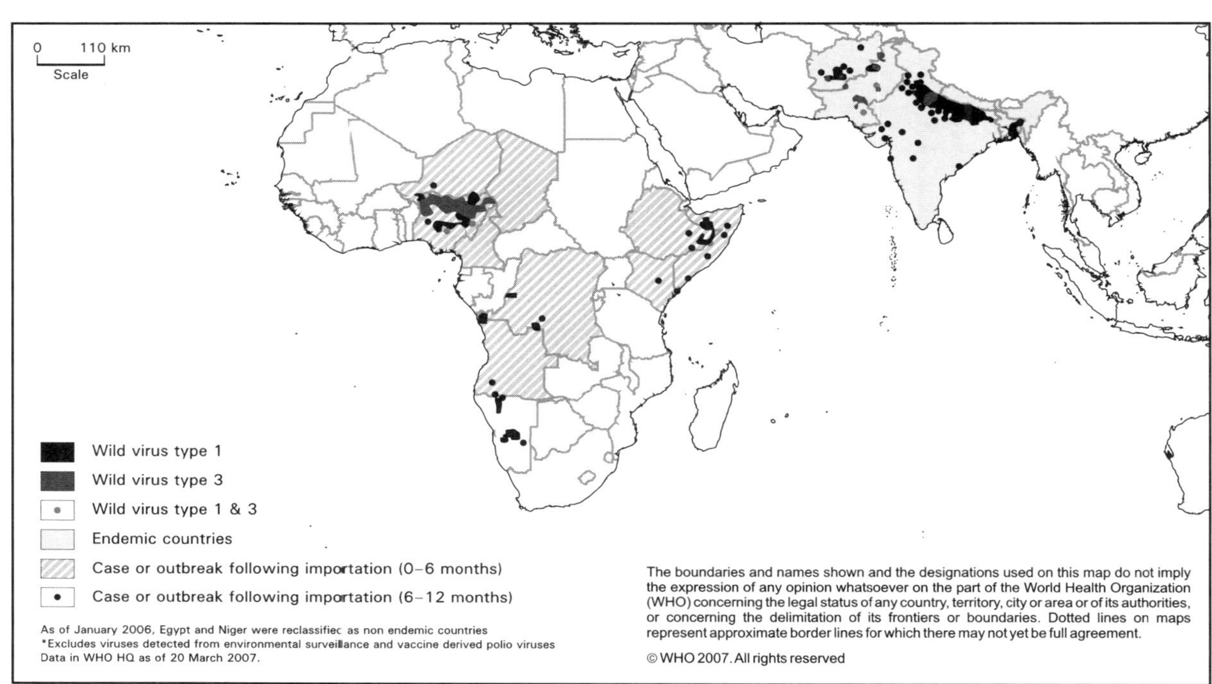

Source: © World Health Organization.

was done by smallpox eradication. Instead, very high vaccination coverage over a large area is needed. Considering this aspect, wide or large scale vaccination campaigns are in progress, from five to nine times in a year in the above mentioned four endemic nations. However, so far, these immunisation activities have failed to interrupt transmission. Why then were efforts in the South American or East Asian programmes successful even with similar epidemiology of 200 sub-clinical infections per one paralysis case? One plausible reason would be that poverty as well as armed conflicts hamper the smooth implementation of the key polio eradication strategies in the remaining Sub-Saharan and South Asian areas.

Of type 1, 2 and 3 wild poliovirus prevalent over the last few decades, type 2 appears to have been eradicated in recent years. The WHO now recommends the use of monovalent OPV type 1 or type 3 in the hope that such vaccine would augment the immunity level in vaccinated populations in epidemic or endemic areas and decrease the occurrence of vaccine associated polio infections, which although infrequent, can cause additional unexpected problems.

The year 2008 will be the twentieth year of the global eradication programme. Eradication, as shown in the definition, must be done by coordinated global efforts. Those nations lacking the ability to stop wild poliovirus transmission in the planned schedule need to be supported to increase their level of work, even provisionally for a short period of time, so that the global time schedule can be met. Otherwise, prolonged or irregular time schedules in certain areas can cause programme fatigue. To provide this support, so far the programme cost has reached US$5 billion as of 2007. With additional funding, it is hoped that the global eradication effort can succeed in achieving the 2008 target. Research on vaccine-derived poliovirus with potential of prolonged transmission is important, which will be discussed elsewhere.

Lastly, as taught by the smallpox eradication experience with research and field studies, to succeed in the polio endgame, intensive research will be needed. For example, as mentioned already, polio has the enormous number of sub-clinical infection: the WHO indicates, one paralysis among 200 sub-clinical infections, the ratio may increase up to 0.1 per cent paralysis among sub-clinical infections.[8] In the polio eradication operation, this pattern of infection hampers the effective surveillance on acute flaccid paralysis surveillance in the programme. What is suspected is that polio virus may be circulating silently and rapidly among new born and unvaccinated age group. In fact, experience shows that more than 70 per cent of polio cases have been in the age group of young children up to thirty-six months of age in recent years. The recommendation to cover all children up to five year of age, if done, will cover this age group, but the programme has not been able to do so, causing a large number of polio in young children. Also it has been said that routine immunisation of OPV at birth and, thereafter three OPV, from four to eleven weeks are important to be combined with the polio immunisation for eradication. The evidence has shown differently. Research is urgently needed to verify above: perhaps meticulous investigations in the selected districts and importantly, prepare the operational manual on how to intensify OPV immunisation of new born and young children, specifically for countries where polio transmission is continuing or exposed to the risk of importation. This research certainly accelerates the progress of polio eradication. Also, such system may serve for other vaccine projects.

Measles eradication, elimination or effective control?

As mentioned, in 1994, the Regional Certification Commission certified that polio transmission in the Americas was interrupted. In the same year, the PAHO launched a measles eradication programme in the region. The measles eradication strategy was developed based on experience in Cuba where measles transmission was successfully interrupted (Figure 6.8, Map 6.5).

[8] Wimmer, "The Test Tube Synthesis of a Chemical called Polio Virus".

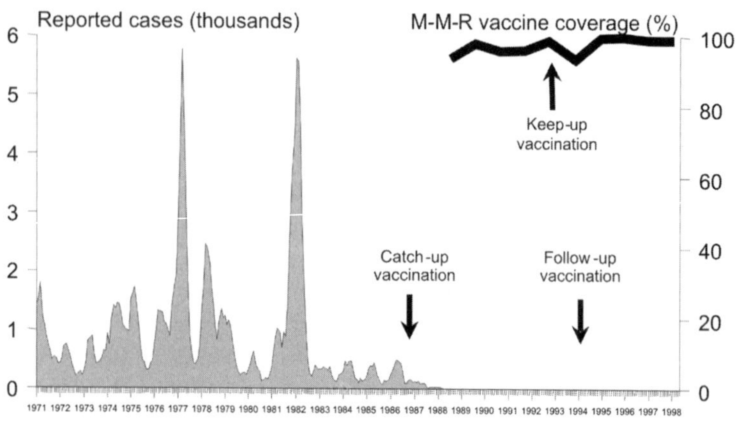

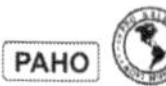

FIGURE 6.8: Reported measles cases by month, Cuba, 1971–98.

Source: Ministry of Health, Cuba.

The measles immunisation strategy consists of:

1. One time overall vaccination of children aged 9 months to 14 years,
2. Thereafter, vaccination of all children aged one to four years every four years—to supplement vaccination of "left-over" children, and
3. Routine vaccination of children aged twelve to fifteen months.[9]

Surveillance is based on reporting and specimen-testing for confirmation of measles viral infection, by a network of WHO approved laboratories. The programme proceeded as planned and around 2000, the indigenous transmission of measles was apparently interrupted in North and South America, leaving occasional importations of measles from other continents and resulting

[9] C. A. de Quadros, B. S. Hersh, A. C. Nogueira, P. A. Carrasco and C. M. Silveria, "Measles Eradication: Experience in the Americas", *Morbidity and Mortality Weekly Supplements* 48 (SU01), Global Disease Elimination as Public Health Strategies, 1999, 57–64.

Map 6.5: Nationwide measles immunisation campaigns, 2004

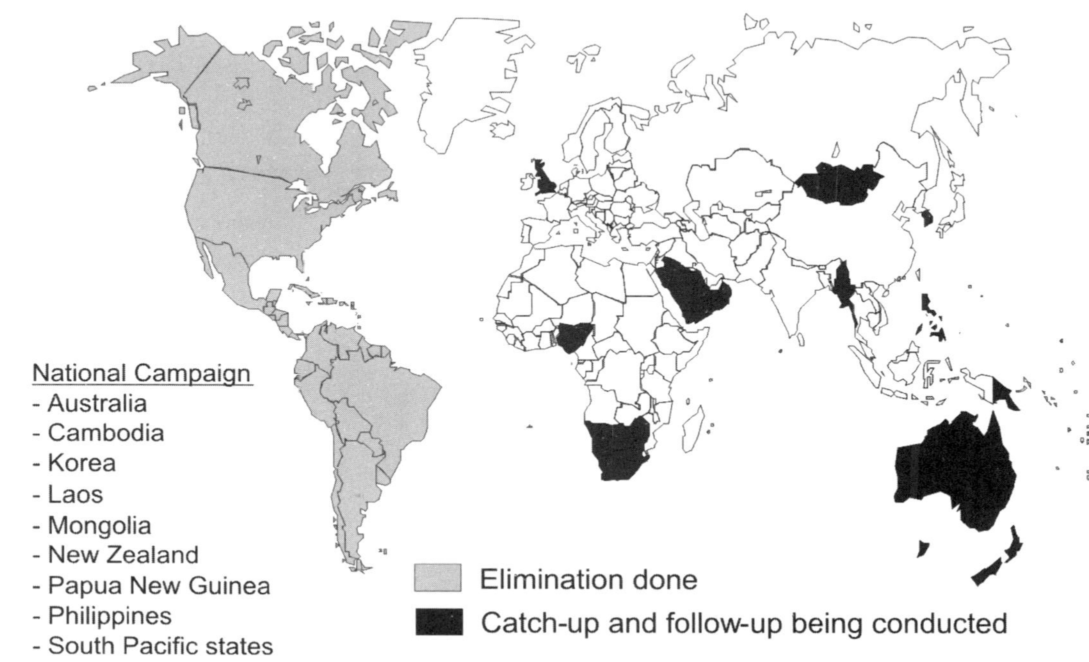

Source: © World Health Organization.

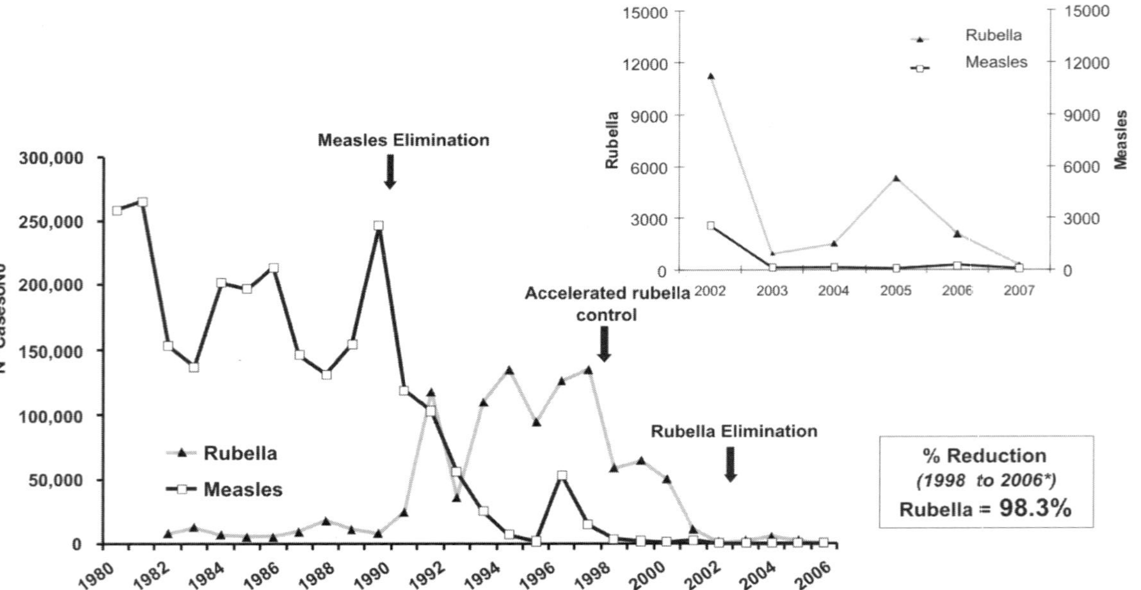

FIGURE 6.9: Impact of rubella and measles elimination strategies: The Americas, 1980–2007*

Note: *Includes rubella and measles cases reported to Pan American Health Organization as of epidemiological week October 2007.

Source: Pan American Health Organization.

outbreaks (Figure 6.9). It is noteworthy that the measles eradication programme has been combined with rubella elimination.

Then, is global eradication of measles feasible? We propose that the answer should be "no". Measles spread is much more rapid than smallpox and polio. This is the reason why the Western Hemisphere, despite the interruption of indigenous transmission, still continues to have frequent importations and resultant outbreaks, as seen in the US. This means, global interruption of measles transmission is only feasible if all the nations on all continents can launch the global strategy more or less at the same time, say within one year. This is almost impossible given today's political conditions. The globalisation era, with its rapid international transport, also increases the need for a synchronised global effort.

Technical issues also affect whether measles can be eradicated. Measles virus is transmittable even before clinical manifestations, which necessitate that measles vaccination coverage as high as 96 per cent and over will be required. This will be difficult to achieve in the resource-limited nations. Also, measles vaccination is highly effective for only nine to twelve months after birth due to maternal antibodies interfering with the vaccine. The duration of maternal antibodies varies, which results in many measles infections in poor countries occurring in infants even before nine months of age.

Therefore, measles eradication may not be achievable with the currently available technologies, but the disease is a good target for an elimination programme. Attempts are being made by many nations, under the WHO's guidance, to stop indigenous measles transmission in as large an area as possible, while improving surveillance and immunisation programmes so that importations can be dealt with effectively. Many countries have now adopted a two-dose measles vaccination schedule: one at twelve months or more after birth and the second before entering primary school. Also, in many nations, EPI includes use of combined vaccine, such as measles/rubella or measles/rubella/mumps.

Eradication of Dracunculiasis

One more disease, dracunculiasis, a parasitic disease occurring in certain regions of Africa and South Asia, has also been the target of an eradication effort since the early 1980s. People entering ponds or water can be infected by the causative agent—larvae. It can be prevented with applying larvacides to infected ponds and also by filtering drinking water in the endemic areas. At present, the situation in Sudan forms a major obstacle to successful eradication (Figure 6.10).

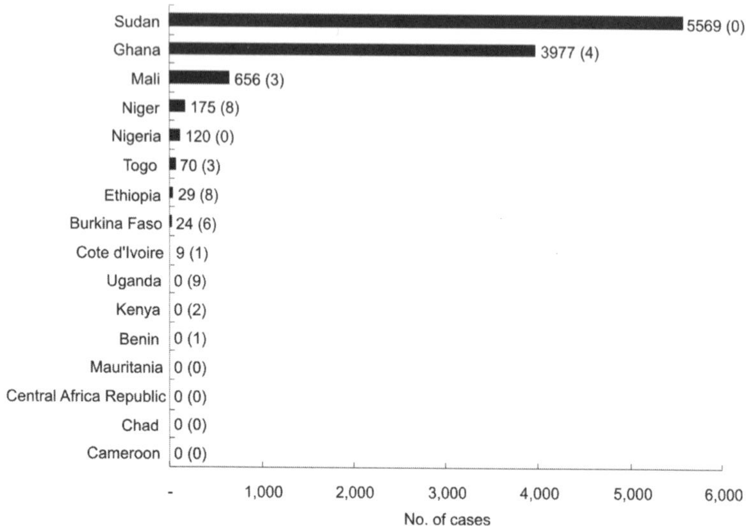

FIGURE 6.10: Distribution of indigenous and imported cases (in parentheses) of dracunculiasis reported in 2005.

Source: World Health Organization, WER No. 24, 16 June 2006.

Conclusions

Despite various efforts made to eradicate diseases, smallpox eradication at present is the only successful one. Major efforts are now being made to eradiate polio with renewed efforts by WHO. [10] Measles has been targeted for elimination or eradication in several

[10] World Health Organization, Press release, "Polio Consultation Reaches Broad Consensus to Complete Polio Eradication", 28 February 2007, http://www.who.int/mediacentre/news/notes/2007/np09/en/index.html.

of WHO's regions, but the feasibility of achieving an eradication goal still needs more research and debate to see if the definition of disease eradication presented in this article can be applied (Table 6.2).

TABLE 6.2: Comparison of features influencing the feasibility of eradication of measles and poliomyelitis, compared with smallpox, in which all features were favourable

	Smallpox	*Measles*	*Poliomyelitis*
Biological features			
Reservoir host in wildlife	No	No	No
Persistent infection occurs	No	Yes[a]	No
Number of serotypes	1	1	3
Antigenically stable	Yes	Yes	Yes
Vaccine			
Effective	Yes	Yes[b]	Yes
Cold chain necessary	No	Yes	Yes
Number of doses	1	2	4
Infectivity in prodromal stage	No	Yes	Yes
Subclinical cases occur	No	No	Yes
Early containment possible	Yes	No	No
Sociopolitical features			
Country-wide elimination achieved	Yes[c]	No	Yes[d]
Financial incentive for assistance	Strong	Week	Week[e]
Records of vaccination required	No – scar	Yes	Yes

a As subacute sclerosing panencephalitis, but since no shedding occurs in this disease it is epidemiologically irrelevant.

b Vaccination is ineffective in the presence of maternal antibody.

c Before the Intensified Smallpox Eradiation Programme commenced, in many countries.

d Before global eradication proposed, in several countries.

e But since 1985 considerable help provided by UNICEF, the World Bank, and others.

Source: David White, O. Fenner and J. Frank, *Medical Virology*, 4th edition (San Diego: Academic Press, 1994).

Currently, poverty is a major component of eradication efforts and an important subject to consider when evaluating the feasibility of disease eradication. While we will consider this topic more fully in other articles, the following summary points are mentioned here.

The intensified smallpox eradication efforts were completed in ten years during which time there was a cold war with the only major armed conflicts, the Indo-Pakistan and the Ethiopia-Somalia wars. They all influenced significantly temporary progress of the global programme, but not the overall progress of the programme. These two time-limited wars were not as serious as the large number of continuing conflicts experienced in endemic areas during polio eradication efforts over the last nineteen years of the programme. Furthermore, a rapidly growing population (currently 6 billion, increasing to 8 billion in the next thirty years), will be coupled with a global widening of inequality, which tends to affect most severely those geographical areas of greatest concern (Table 6.3).[11]

TABLE 6.3: Poverty and diseases: Number of deaths under five years of age, 2003

Area	Population	AIDS	Percentage	Diarrhoea	Percentage	ARI	Percentage	Malaria	Percentage
Europe	50	1	0.3	35	2.0	32	1.6	0	0.0
Americas	77	6	1.9	51	2.9	54	2.7	1	0.1
Western Pacific	130	3	0.9	178	10.1	137	6.8	1	0.1
Africa*	110	285	88.8	701	39.8	924	45.5	802	94.0
South East Asia*	178	22	6.9	552	31.3	590	29.1	12	1.4
East Mediterranean	68	4	1.2	245	13.9	292	14.4	37	4.3
Total	613	321	100.0	1,762	100.0	2,029	100.0	853	100.0

Note: Population is that of children under five years of age in 100,000.

* Of 1.1 billion persons with $1.08 per day worldwide, 314 million (29 per cent) and 428 million (40 per cent) persons from Sub-Saharan Africa and from South Asia respectively in 2001.

Source: World Health Organization, *The World Health Report 2005: Make Every Mother and Child Count* (Geneva: World Health Organization, 2005); The World Bank, *World Development Indicators 2004* (Washington DC: The World Bank, 2004).

[11] William Easterly, "The Future of Western Assistance", in *The White Man's Burden: Why the West's Efforts to Aid the Rest Have Done So Much Ill and So Little Good* (London: Penguin Books, 2006), 367–84.

Disease eradication presents a very special case for international cooperation which is necessary for it to succeed. Unless some solutions to the abovementioned problems can be worked out, disease eradication will be increasingly difficult in the twenty-first century. 'Peace' is a prerequisite for disease eradication, but implementing this simple and clean word is proving more difficult than stating it.

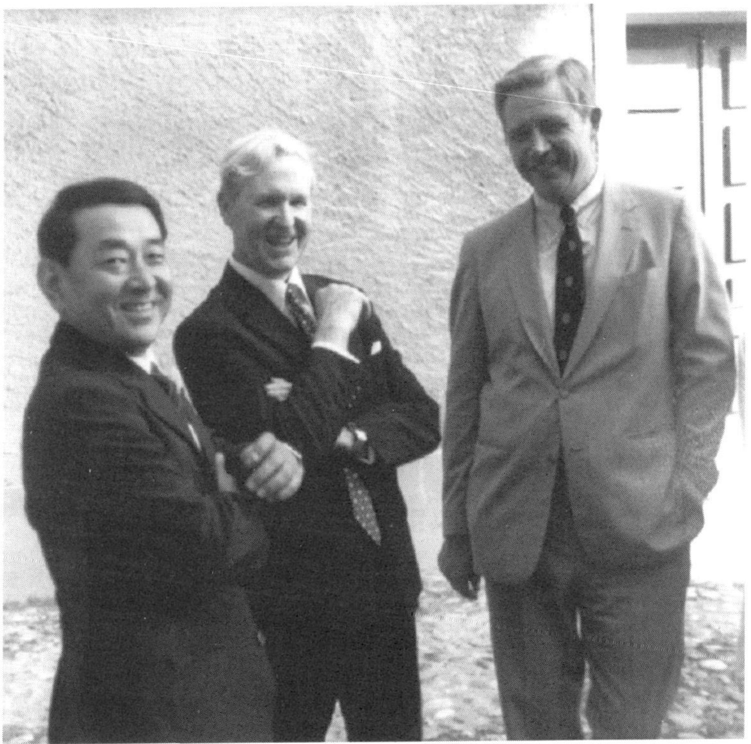

FIGURE 6.11: D. A. Henderson, Frank Fenner and Isao Arita at the Nairobi International Centre where the commission meeting for the certification of smallpox eradication was held in late 1979.

Source: Photograph provided by the author.

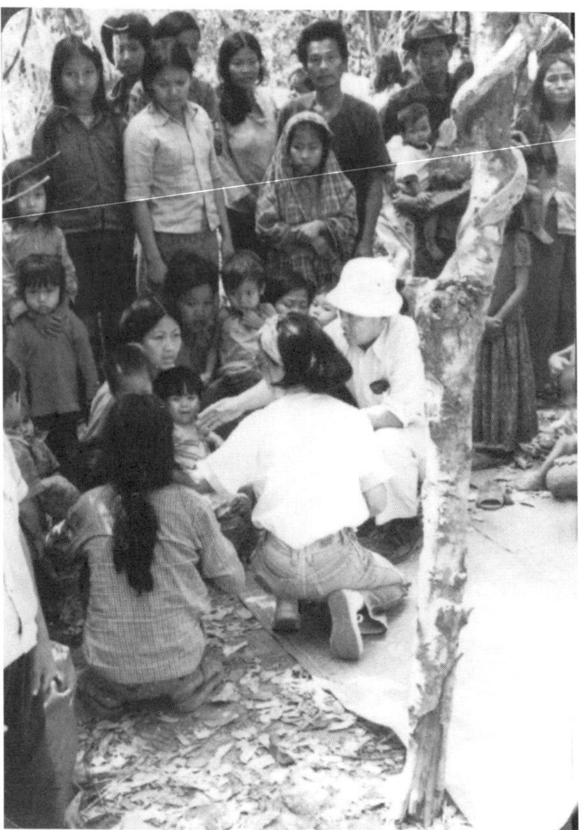

FIGURE 6.12: Dr Isao Arita working on the Cambodia Burma border region. Mothers were very keen to take care of their children and in an announcement that WHO doctors were coming and large number arrived. We were usually happy to take care of their general health in addition to smallpox surveillance and often prescribed vitamins.

Source: Photograph provided by the author.

Bibliography

Arita, I., J. Wickett and F. Fenner. "Impact of Population Density on Immunization Programmes". *Journal of Hygiene* 96, 1986, 459–66.

Basu, R. N. "Smallpox Surveillance Status in India". *Journal of Communicable Diseases* 6, 1974, 177–83.

Basu, R. N., Z. Jezek and N. A. Ward. *The Eradication of Smallpox from India.* New Delhi: World Health Organization, 1979.

Bhattacharya, Sanjoy. *Expunging Variola: The Control and Eradication of Smallpox in India 1947–1977.* Hyderabad: Orient Longman, 2006.

Breman, J. G. "Monkeypox: An Emerging Infection for Humans?" In *Emerging Infections 4*, ed. W. M. Scheld, W. A. Craig and J. M. Hughes, 45–67. Washington DC: American Society for Microbiology, 2000.

Breman, J. G. and I. Arita. "The Confirmation and Maintenance of Smallpox Eradication". *New England Journal of Medicine* 303, 1980, 1263–73.

Breman, J. G., A. B. Alecaut and J. M. Lane. "Smallpox in the Republic of Guinea, West Africa: I. History and Epidemiology". *American Journal of Tropical Medicine and Hygiene* 26, 1977, 756–64.

Breman, J. G., A. B. Alecaut, D. R. Malberg, R. S. Charter and J. M. Lane. "Smallpox in the Republic of Guinea, West Africa: II. Eradication Using Mobile Teams". *American Journal of Tropical Medicine and Hygiene* 26, 1977, 765–74.

Breman, J. G., and D. A. Henderson. "Diagnosis and Management of Smallpox". *New England Journal of Medicine* 346, 2002, 300–8.

Breman, J. G., E. Coffi, K. R.Bomba-Ire, S. O. Foster and K. L. Herrman. "Evaluation of a Measles-smallpox Vaccination Campaign by a Sero-epidemiologic Method". *American Journal of Epidemiology* 102, 1975, 564–71.

Breman, J. G., M. V. Kalisa-Ruti, M. V. Steniowski, E. Zanotto, A. I. Gromyko and I. Arita. "Human Monkeypox. 1970–79". *Bulletin of the World Health Organization* 58, 1980, 165–82.

Brilliant, Larry, and Girija Brilliant. "Death for a Killer Disease: How an Army of Samaritans Drove Smallpox from the Earth". *Quest Magazine*, May/June 1978.

Brilliant, Larry. *The Management of Smallpox Eradication in India.* Ann Arbor: University of Michigan Press, 1985.

De Quadros, C. A., B. S. Hersh, A. C. Nogueira, P. A. Carrasco, and C. M. Silveria. "Measles Eradication: Experience in the Americas". *Morbidity and Mortality Weekly Report Supplements* 48 (SU01), Global Disease Elimination and Eradication as Public Health Strategies, 1999, 57–64.

Dowdle, Walter R. and Donald R. Hopkins, eds. *The Eradication of Infectious Diseases: Report of the Dahlem Workshop on the Eradication of Infectious Diseases, Berlin March 16–22, 1997.* West Sussex: John Wiley & Sons, 1998.

Duffy, J., ed. *Ventures in World Health: The Memoirs of Fred Lowe Soper.* Washington DC: Pan American Health Organization, 1977.

Dutta, M., et al. "Lessons Learnt from the Intensified Campaign against Smallpox in India and their Applicability to other National Health Programmes". *Journal of Communicable Diseases* 7, 1975, 209–13.

Easterly, William. "The Future of Western Assistance". In *The White Man's Burden: Why the West's Efforts to Aid the Rest Have Done So Much Ill and So Little Good*, ed. William Easterly, 367–84. London: Penguin Books, 2006.

Esposito, J. J., J. F. Obijeski and J. H. Nakano. "Serological Relatedness of Monkeypox, Variola, and Vaccinia Viruses". *Journal of Medical Virology* 1, 1977, 35–47.

Farid, M. A. "The Malaria Programme: From Euphoria to Anarchy". *World Health Forum* 1, 1980, 15.

Fasquelle, R. and A. Fasquelle. "A Propos de l'Histoire de la Lutte Contre la Variole dans les Pays d'Afrique Francophone". *Bulletin de la Société de Pathologie Exotique* 64, 1971, 734–56.

Fenner F., D. A. Henderson, I. Arita, Z. Jezek and I. D. Ladnyi. *Smallpox and its Eradication*. Geneva: World Health Organization, 1988.

Foege W. "Can Smallpox Be as Simple as 1–2–3?" *Washington Post*, 29 December 2002.

Foege, W. H., J. D. Millar and D. A. Henderson. "Smallpox Eradication in West and Central Africa". *Bulletin of the World Health Organization* 52, 1975, 209–22.

Foege, W. H., J. D. Millar and J. M. Lane, "Selective Epidemiological Control in Smallpox Eradicaiton". *American Journal of Epidemiology* 94, 1971, 311–15.

Foster, S. O., and E. A. Smith. "The Epidemiology of Smallpox in Nigeria". *Journal of the Nigeria Medical Association* 7, 1970, 41–45.

Foster, S. O. *Persistence of Facial Scars of Smallpox in West African Populations*. Geneva: World Health Organization, 1970.

Gelfand, H. M. "A Critical Examination of the Indian Smallpox Eradication Programme". *American Journal of Public Health* 56, 1966, 1634–51.

Gelfand, H. M. and D. A. Henderson. "A Programme for Smallpox Eradication and Measles Control throughout West Africa". *Journal of International Health* 2, 1966, 24–33.

Greenough, Paul. "Intimidation, Coercion and Resistance in the Final Stages of the South Asian Smallpox Eradication Campaign, 1973–1975", *Social Science and Medicine* 41, no. 5, 1995, 633–45.

Henderson, D. A. "Report on a Visit to the Smallpox Eradication Programme, India", World Health Organization, SEA/SPX [restricted], World Health Organization, New Delhi, June 1972.

———. "The Deliberate Extinction of a Species". *Proceedings of the American Philosophical Society* 126, 1982, 461–71.

———. "Keynote Address". *Bulletin of the World Health Organization* 76, supplement 2, 1998, 14–16.

———. "Eradication: Lessons from the Past". *Bulletin of the World Health Organization* 76, supplement 2, 1998, 17–21.

———. *Smallpox: The Death of a Disease. The Inside Story of Eradicating a Worldwide Killer*. Amherst, NY: Prometheus Books, 2009.

Henderson, R. H. and M. Yekpe. "Smallpox Transmission in Southern Dahomey: A Study of a Village Outbreak". *American Journal of Epidemiology* 90, no. 5, 1969, 423–28.

Henderson, R. H., H. Davis, D. I. Eddins and W. Foege. "Assessment of Vaccination Coverage, Vaccination Scar rates, and Smallpox Scarring in Five Areas of West Africa". *Bulletin of the World Health Organization* 48, 1973, 183–94.

Hopkins, D. R. *Princes and Peasants: Smallpox in History*. Chicago: University of Chicago Press, 1983.

———. *The Greatest Killer: Smallpox in History.* Chicago: University of Chicago Press, 2002.

Hopkins, D. R., J. M. Lane, E. C. Cummings and J. D. Millar. "Smallpox in Sierra Leone: I. Epidemiology". *American Journal of Tropical Medicine and Hygiene* 20, 1971, 689–96.

———. "Smallpox in Sierra Leone: II. The 1968–69 Eradication Program". *American Journal of Tropical Medicine and Hygiene* 20, 1971, 697–704.

Hopkins, D. R., J. M. Lane, E. C. Cummings and J. D. Millar. "Two Funeral-associated Smallpox Outbreaks in Sierra Leone". *American Journal of Epidemiology* 94, 1971, 341–47.

Imperato, P. J. "The Use of Markets as Vaccination Sites in the Mali Republic". *American Journal of Tropical Medicine and Hygiene* 72, 1969, 8–13.

———. "Observations on Variolation Practices in Mali". *Tropical and Geographical Medicine* 26, 1974, 429–40.

———. "Nomads of the West African Sahel and the Delivery of Health Services to Them". *Social Science and Medicine* 8, 1974, 443–57.

Imperato, P. J., O. Sow and B. Fofana. "Mass Campaigns and Their Comparative Operational Costs for Nomadic and Sedentary Populations in the Republic of Mali". *Tropical and Geographical Medicine* 25, 1973, 516–22.

Ježek, Z. and F. Fenner. *Human Monkeypox.* Basel: Karger, 1988.

Joarder, A. K., D. Tarantola and J. Tulloch. *The Eradication of Smallpox from Bangladesh.* New Delhi: World Health Organization South-East Asia Regional Office, 1980.

Lapeyssonie, L. "Jamot parmi nous". *Medécine Tropicale*, 1963, 461–69.

Le Fanu, W. R. *A Bio-Bibliography of Edward Jenner, 1749-1823*. London: Harvey and Blythe, 1951.

Macaulay, T. B. *The History of England from the Accession of James II*. London: J. M. Dent & Sons, 1800.

Maury, C. *Folk Origins in Indian Art*. New York: Columbia University Press, 1969.

Millar, J. D., R. R. Roberto, H. Wulff, H. A. Wenner and D. A. Henderson. "Smallpox Vaccination by Intradermal Jet Injection: 1. Introduction, Background, and Results of Pilot Studies". *Bulletin of the World Health Organization* 41, 1969, 749–60.

Nakano, J. H., Albert Balows, William J. Hauster Jr. and Joseph P. Truant. "Smallpox, Monkeypox, Vaccinia, and Whitepox Viruses". In *Manual of Clinical Microbiology*, ed. E. H. Lennette and J. P. Truant, 810–22. 3rd edition. Washington DC: American Society for Microbiology, 1980.

Neff, J. M., J. D. Millar, R. R. Roberto and H. Wulff. "Smallpox Vaccination by Intradermal Jet Injection: 3. Evaluation in a Well-vaccinated Population". *Bulletin of the World Health Organization* 41, 1969, 771–78.

Ogden, H. G. *CDC and the Smallpox Crusade*. Washington DC: US Department of Health and Human Services, Public Health Service, Centers for Disease Control, 1987.

Richet, P. "L'histoire et l'oeuvre de l'O.C.C.G.E. en Afrique occidentale francophone". *Transactions of the Royal Society of Tropical Medicine and Hygiene* 59, 1965, 234–54.

Roberto, R. R., H. Wulff and J. D. Millar. "Smallpox Vaccination by Jet Injection: 2. Cutaneous and Serological Responses to Primary Vaccination in Children". *Bulletin of the World Health Organization* 41, 1969, 761–69.

Scholtens, R. G., R. L. Kaiser and A. D. Langmuir. "An Epidemiologic Examination of the Strategy of Malaria Eradication". *International Journal of Epidemiology* 1, 1972, 15–24.

Saliou, P. and J. G. Breman. "Une Mallette Pour la Surveillance Epidémiologique de la Variole, du Cholera et de la Fièvre Jaune:

Note de Présentation". *Bulletin Sociéte Pathologie Exotique et des Filiales* 69, 1976, 398–411.

Saliou, P., J. L. Rey, J. G. Breman and P. Stoekel. "Une année d'utilisation en Haute Volta d'une mallette pour la surveillance du cholera, de la fièvre jaune et de la variole". *Bulletin Sociéte Pathologie Exotique et des Filiales* 70, 1977, 544–52.

Schnur, A. "WHO Epidemiologist Tour Diary". Unpublished, Dhaka, 1975

Tekeste, Yemane, Alebachew Hailu, C. do Amaral, P. R. Arbani, O. Ismail, L. N. Khodakevich and N. A. Ward. *Smallpox Eradication in Ethiopia*. Brazzaville: World Health Organization, 1984.

The Report of the Royal Commission on Vaccination. London, 1896.

Thompson, D. and W. Foege. *Faith Tabernacle Smallpox Epidemic Abakaliki, Nigeria.* Geneva: World Health Organization, 1968.

Waddy, B. B. "Rural Health Services in the Tropics and the Training of Medical Auxiliaries for Them". *Transactions of the Royal Society of Tropical Medical Hygiene* 57, 1963, 384–91.

White, David, O. Fenner and J. Frank, *Medical Virology*, 4th edition. San Diego: Academic Press, 1994.

Wimmer, Eckard. "The Test-tube Synthesis of a Chemical called Poliovirus". *European Molecular Biology Organization Report* 7, special issue, 2006, S3–S9.

World Health Organization. "Proposals for World-wide Campaigns: Smallpox". Official Records of the World Health Organization, no. 48, 1953.

——. *The Global Eradiation of Smallpox: Final Report of the Global Commission for the Certification of Smallpox Eradiation.* Geneva: World Health Organization, 1980.

——. Press release. "Polio Consultation Reaches Broad Consensus to Complete Polio Eradication". 28 February 2007, http://www.who.int/mediacentre/news/notes/2007/np09/en/index.html.

Yekutiel, P. "Lessons from the Big Eradication Campaigns". *World Health Forum* 2, no. 4, 1981, 470–71.

Contributors

Isao Arita, M.D. PhD began work in the Japanese Ministry of Health. In 1962 he became involved with the smallpox programme at the WHO Regional Office for Africa and in 1964 was transferred to the Virus Unit of the WHO headquarters. In 1967 he joined the new unit for smallpox eradication where he worked until 1985. From 1977 to 1985 he was appointed as the Chief of the unit having worked with many WHO and national staff, specifically for the last fight in the Horn of Africa, the certifications for 1980 WHO declaration of smallpox eradication and preparation for post-eradication strategy. He currently continues his involvement in WHO initiatives, advises on WHO research committees and variola and polio eradication initiatives.
Email: oiarita@ms2.infobears.ne.jp

Sanjoy Bhattacharya leaves his position as Reader at the Wellcome Trust Centre for the History of Medicine at UCL on the 30 September 2010, after which he joins the Department of History at the University of York, as a Reader in History, on the 1 October 2010. Dr Bhattacharya specialises in the history of nineteenth and twentieth century South Asia, as well as the history of international and global health programmes deployed in the South Asian subcontinent and beyond. Dr Bhattacharya's current work examines the structures and workings of health programmes sponsored and managed by agencies of the UN, such as the WHO; the development of public health and medical institutions at all levels of national and local administration; and the diversity of social and political responses to state-medicine. He is also developing an

active research programme dealing with the absorption of medical professionals from across South Asia, with particular reference to India and Sri Lanka, into the UK's National Health Service.
Email: joygeeta@hotmail.com

Joel G. Breman, M.D., D.T.P.H., F.I.D.S.A., is Senior Scientific Adviser at the Fogarty International Center of the US National Institutes of Health. Dr Breman's recent research has defined the considerable burden of malaria and policies and practices to conquer this disease. Dr Breman worked in Guinea on smallpox eradication and measles control (1967–69); in Burkina Faso at the Organisation for Coordination and Cooperation in the Control of the Major Endemic Diseases (1972–76) where he was Chief of the Epidemiology Section; and, at the WHO, Geneva (1977–80), where he was responsible for coordinating orthopoxvirus research and the certification of smallpox eradication. In 1976, in the Democratic Republic of Congo (formerly Zaire), Dr Breman investigated the first outbreak of Ebola haemorrhagic fever as part of an international commission. Following the confirmation of smallpox eradication in 1980, Dr Breman returned to the US Centers for Disease Control and Prevention, where he began work on the epidemiology and control of malaria. He joined the Fogarty Inter-national Center in 1995 and has been Director of the International Training and Research Programme in Emerging Infectious Diseases and other institutional strengthening programmes in low-income countries. Since 2001, he has been Co-managing Editor of the Disease Control Priorities Project (www.dcp2.org) and lead editor of three volumes of articles on "the intolerable burden of malaria" published as supplements to the *American Journal of Tropical Medicine and Hygiene* (www.ajtmh.org).
Email: jbreman@nih.gov

Larry Brilliant M.D. MPH is the President of Skoll Global Threats Fund which works on pandemics, water, climate change, nuclear non-proliferation and conflict in the Middle East. He was formerly VP of Google and executive director of Google.org. Dr Brilliant is board-certified in preventive medicine. He was a WHO medical officer part of the SEARO smallpox eradication

team and lived in India for ten years. He is the author of the book "The Management of Smallpox in India" (University of Michigan Press, 1980). He taught epidemiology and international health at University of Michigan and in 1978 he founded the Seva Foundation, which works in dozens of countries around the world, primarily to eliminate preventable and curable blindness. In 2006, he won the TED prize. In 2008, TIME magazine named him one of the 20 most influential scientists and thinkers.
Email: larrybrilliant@gmail.com

Corrie White Conrad joined Google in early 2007 as a Researcher with an initial focus on malaria and the eradication of smallpox. She is currently a Programme Manager with Google's philanthropic branch, Google.org, where she manages Global health projects like Google Flu trends, a tool that uses aggregated search queries for tracking influenza in near real-time. Previously, Corrie was a Programme Officer with the Clinton Foundation HIV/AIDS Initiative in Rwanda where she worked closely with the government to support the scale-up of pediatric HIV/AIDS care and treatment. She also worked with a variety of non-profit organisations to support international education in Zimbabwe, India and Rwanda. Corrie was a Morehead Scholar at the University of North Carolina at Chapel Hill and did her graduate work at Princeton University.
Email: cconrad@google.com

D. A. Henderson is a Distinguished Scholar at the Center for Biosecurity of the University of Pittsburgh Medical Center and a Professor of Public Health and Medicine at the University of Pittsburgh. He is Dean Emeritus and Professor at the Johns Hopkins School of Public Health and a Founding Director (1998) of the Johns Hopkins Center for Civilian Biodefense Strategies. Dr Henderson's previous positions include: Associate Director of the Office of Science and Technology Policy, Executive Office of the President (1990–93); Dean of the Faculty of the Johns Hopkins School of Public Health (1977–90); and Director of the WHO's global smallpox eradication campaign (1966–77). He is the author of the book, *Smallpox, Death of a Disease* (2009) which vividly documents

the unprecedented challenges and international collaborations that account for its total eradication.
Email: dahzero@aol.com

Sharon Messenger joined the Wellcome Trust Centre for the History of Medicine at UCL in 1999 where she holds the position of Senior Research Assistant. She co-edited (with Michael Neve) Charles Darwin's *Autobiographies* for Penguin Classics (2002) and more recently completed an edition of Darwin's *Expression of the Emotions in Man and Animals* (with Joe Cain), also for Penguin Classics 2009. She continues to work on the Wellcome-funded Livingstone Online project which edits the medical and scientific correspondence of David Livingstone (www.livingstoneonline.ucl.ac.uk). She worked closely with Sanjoy Bhattacharya on the *History of Social Determinants of Health: Global Histories, Contemporary Debates* (2007) and also *Social Determinants of Health: Assessing Theory, Policy and Practice* (with Sanjoy Bhattacharya and Caroline Overy) in 2010 both published by Orient BlackSwan.
Email: s.messenger@ucl.ac.uk

Miyuki Nakane obtained a Bachelor of Applied Science (Environmental Health), from Flinders University, Australia in 1998. From 1998 to 2008, she worked for the Agency for Cooperation in International Health (ACIH) and was in charge of the research on how to develop and utilize the sentinel-based surveillance on emerging and re-emerging diseases, AGSnet (Alumni for Global Surveillance network). In 2000 and 2001 she participated in Global Outbreak Alert and Response Network meetings in WHO headquarters, also, planning and managing the training courses on infectious diseases in collaboration with Japan International Cooperation Agency (JICA), targeting child health and vaccine preventable diseases. In 2009, she joined Kumamoto University and is currently working in the Finance Department.
E-mail: miux@jn2.so-net.ne.jp

Ciro de Quadros, M.D., M.P.H., is the Executive Vice-President of the Albert B. Sabin Vaccine Institute in Washington DC. A pioneer in developing effective strategies for smallpox surveillance

and containment, Dr de Quadros served as the WHO's chief epidemiologist for smallpox eradication in Ethiopia during the 1970s. Following the global eradication of smallpox, he became the Regional Immunisation Advisor and then the Director of the Division of Vaccines and Immunisation for the Pan American Health Organization, for whom he successfully directed efforts to eradicate poliomyelitis and measles from the Western Hemisphere. Dr de Quadros is the technical advisor on vaccines and immunisation for the International Pediatric Association and serves as the Chairperson of the PAHO's Technical Advisory Group on Vaccines and Immunisation. He is a faculty member at the Johns Hopkins School of Hygiene and Public Health and the School of Medicine at George Washington University.
Email: ciro.dequadros@sabin.org

Alan Schnur is a former WHO staff member. Following his work in the smallpox eradication programme in Ethiopia, India, Bangladesh, Somalia and Geneva (1971–1978), he worked in the Expanded Programme on Immunisation units in two WHO regional offices: South-East Asia and the Western Pacific (1982–1994). He was a member of the Polio Eradication Task Force at the Regional Office for the Western Pacific. During his assignment at the WHO country office in China (1994–2003), he worked on polio eradication and disease surveillance and response issues, including the response to the Severe Acute Respiratory Syndrome (SARS) outbreak in 2003. Mr Schnur's last assignment before retirement was with the evaluation unit at the WHO headquarters in Geneva (2003–2010). His interests include sustaining awareness about the management successes of the smallpox eradication programme, particularly the establishment of a culture of evaluation at all levels of the programme.
Email: schnurah@gmail.com

Index